NUTRITIONAL FACTORS IN HYPERTENSION

CONTEMPORARY ISSUES IN CLINICAL NUTRITION

Series Editor
Richard S. Rivlin, M.D.

Contemporary Issues in Clinical Nutrition Volumes 1–7, were published by Churchill Livingstone, Inc.

NUTRITIONAL FACTORS IN HYPERTENSION

SECTION A: SELECTED NUTRIENTS

Editors

Herbert Langford

Endocrinology and Hypertension Division
University of Mississippi Medical Center
Jackson, Mississippi

Barbara Levine

Nutrition Information Center
Memoral Sloan-Kettering Cancer Center and
The New York Hospital-Cornell University Medical
College
New York, New York

SECTION B: EMERGING ISSUES RELATED TO CALCIUM INTAKE

Editor

Leon Ellenbogen

Nutritional Sciences
Lederle Laboratories
Pearl River, New York

ALAN R. LISS, INC. · NEW YORK

Library of Congress Cataloging-in-Publication Data

Nutritional factors in hypertension.
        p.   cm. -- (Contemporary issues in clinical nutrition ; v. 12)
    Includes bibliographical references.
    Contents: section A. Selected nutrients / editors, Herbert
Langford, Barbara Levine -- section B. Emerging issues related to
calcium intake / editor, Leon Ellenbogen.
    ISBN 0-471-56233-5
    1. Hypertension--Nutritional aspects. 2. Calcium--Metabolism.
I. Langford, Herbert G. II. Levine, Barbara Stevenson.
III. Ellenbogen, Leon. IV. Series.
RC685.H8N88   1989
616.1'32--dc20   89-12186
                                                           CIP

Contents

Contributors

Richard D. Bukoski, Division of Nephrology and Hypertension, Department of Medicine, Department of Physiology, Oregon Health Sciences University, Portland, OR 97201 **[107]**

Tilman B. Drüeke, INSERM U. 90, Département de Néphrologie, Hôpital Necker, Paris, France **[155]**

Leon Ellenbogen, Nutritional Sciences, Lederle Laboratories, Pearl River, NY 10965 **[ix]**

Bonita Falkner, Department of Pediatrics, Hahnemann University, Philadelphia, PA 19102 **[51]**

Howard S. Friedman, Downstate Medical Center, State University of New York, The Brooklyn Hospital, Brooklyn, NY 11201 **[35]**

Linda M. Gerber, Cardiovascular Center, Cornell University Medical College, New York, NY 10021 **[67]**

Lynne C. Harlan, University of Michigan School of Public Health, University of Michigan Medical School, Ann Arbor, MI 48109; present address: Division of Cancer Prevention and Control, National Cancer Institute, Bethesda, MD 48109 **[175]**

William R. Harlan, University of Michigan School of Medicine, University of Michigan Medical School, Ann Arbor, MI 48109; present address: Division of Epidemiology and Clinical Applications, National Heart, Lung, and Blood Institute, Bethesda, MD 20892 **[175]**

Bernard Lamport, Department of Epidemiology and Social Medicine, Albert Einstein College of Medicine, Bronx, NY 10461 **[17]**

Herbert Langford, Endocrinology and Hypertension Division, University of Mississippi Medical Center, Jackson, MI 39216-4505 **[ix]**

Barbara Levine, Nutrition Information Center, Memoral Sloan-Kettering Cancer Center and The New York Hospital-Cornell University Medical College, New York, NY 10021 **[ix]**

David A. McCarron, Division of Nephrology and Hypertension, Department of Medicine, Department of Physiology, Oregon Health Sciences University, Portland, OR 97201 **[99,107]**

Suzanne H. Michel, Department of Pediatrics, Hahnemann University, Philadelphia, PA 19102 **[51]**

The numbers in brackets are the opening page numbers of the contributors' articles.

Thomas G. Pickering, Cardiovascular Center, The New York Hospital-Cornell Medical Center, New York, NY 10021 **[3]**

Andrew I. Rabinowitz, Department of Pediatrics, Hahnemann University, Philadelphia, PA 19102 **[51]**

James R. Sowers, Division of Endocrinology and Hypertension, Wayne State University, Detroit, MI 48202, and VA Medical Center, Allen Park, MI 48101 **[131]**

C. Swencionis, Department of Epidemiology and Social Medicine, Albert Einstein College of Medicine & Ferknauf Graduate School, Bronx, NY 10461 **[79]**

Frank F. Vincenzi, Department of Pharmacology, University of Washington, Seattle, WA 98195 **[145]**

Sylvia Wassertheil-Smoller, Department of Epidemiology and Social Medicine, Albert Einstein College of Medicine, Bronx, NY 10461 **[17]**

J. Wylie-Rosett, Department of Epidemiology and Social Medicine, Albert Einstein College of Medicine, Bronx, NY 10461 **[79]**

Eric W. Young, Division of Nephrology and Hypertension, Department of Medicine, Department of Physiology, Oregon Health Sciences University, Portland, OR 97201 **[107]**

Michael B. Zemel, Department of Nutrition and Food Science and Division of Endocrinology and Hypertension, Wayne State University, Detroit, MI 48202, and VA Medical Center, Allen Park, MI 48101 **[131]**

Preface

In the U.S., hypertension is a public health problem of enormous magnitude. There is now substantial evidence to suggest that diet has a major influence on the prevention and treatment of hypertension. Nutrition intervention, currently recommended as part of the treatment for established hypertension, may help with prevention as well.

Of the many dietary factors that may affect blood pressure, obesity, sodium, and alcohol have been well substantiated. There is also considerable research on the effects of other dietary factors that include calcium, potassium, magnesium, linoleic acid, caffeine, omega 3-fatty acids, and dietary fat and fiber.

This volume can be divided into two parts. The first six chapters serve as an overview of nutritional influences on the pathophysiology of hypertension. Included are topics related to the epidemiology of nutrition and hypertension, effects of alcohol and hypertension, nutritional issues related to childhood hypertension, and a dietary approach to the management of hypertension. The last six chapters deal with the issue of the role of calcium in hypertension. Dr. McCarron's pioneering work has led many investigators to pursue this area. There is increasing evidence that dietary calcium and regulation of overall calcium metabolism may be a pathological link in the genesis of hypertension in many individuals.

There is rapid growth of knowledge and interest in the area of nutrition and hypertension. We hope that some of the questions and problems posed in these chapters may soon by resolved.

Barbara Levine
Leon Ellenbogen

Section A:

SELECTED NUTRIENTS

Nutritional Factors in Hypertension
© *1990 Alan R. Liss, Inc., pages 3–16*

1

Nutritional Influences on the Pathophysiology of Hypertension

Thomas G. Pickering, M.D., D. Phil.

INTRODUCTION

Essential hypertension is most probably the end result of the interaction of a number of factors, both environmental and genetic. Of the environmental factors, two of the three that have received the most attention (sodium intake, weight gain, and psychosocial stress) are nutritional in origin. The role of weight gain is well accepted, while the other two remain highly controversial as etiological factors. At the present time, the evidence would favor the view that these factors may contribute to the development of hypertension in a minority of individuals who are particularly susceptible to their influence. This susceptibility is currently being studied most intensively for the role of sodium intake, and may be genetically determined.

This chapter will review the mechanism by which the two major nutritional influences on blood pressure, obesity and sodium intake, may exert their effects. The pathophysiological role of other nutritional factors such as potassium, divalent cations, and alcohol are reviewed elsewhere.

PATHOPHYSIOLOGY OF OBESITY AND HYPERTENSION

Numerous epidemiological studies have documented the association between obesity and hypertension [13], and there is also abundant evidence that

From the New York Hospital-Cornell University Medical College, 525 East 68th Street, Starr-4, New York, NY 10021.

weight loss can lower blood pressure in such patients, as exemplified by the recent study of MacMahon et al. [47].

Hemodynamic Factors

The principal hemodynamic changes associated with obesity are an increased cardiac output and blood volume, according to some investigators [51], although others have reported both of these to be normal [58]. In this context, the basal metabolic rate is of great interest: on the one hand, a decreased metabolic rate might be a possible cause of obesity; on the other, an increased cardiac output might be expected if the metabolic rate was increased. The consensus is that it is raised little if at all [29]. When cardiac output is elevated, it may be attributed to an increased preload [20,32]. Left ventricular hypertrophy is relatively common. (Messerli et al., 1984) [50].

In patients who have both hypertension and obesity, the main change is that peripheral resistance is elevated in addition to cardiac output [50].

Hormonal Factors

There appears to be no consistent differences in plasma renin or aldosterone between normal weight and obese subjects, whether or not they are hypertensive, although plasma catecholamines tend to be elvated [7,66,68]. A more consistent link between obesity and blood pressure may be hyperinsulinemia: Three studies have shown correlations between serum insulin and blood pressure in obese subjects [5,42,48]. Such hyperinsulinemia could contribute to the elevation of pressure by at least two mechanisms: first, insulin has a sodium-retaining effect on the kidney and second, it may raise plasma norepinephrine and other indices of sympathetic nervous activity [64]. These effects are independent of blood glucose levels.

CARDIOVASCULAR AND HORMONAL EFFECTS OF CHANGES IN CALORIC INTAKE

Fasting lowers blood pressure, and this is associated with diminished plasma catecholamines [25,31,82]. Conversely, overfeeding sucrose to spontaneously hypertensive rats raises blood pressure [81] and sympathetic nervous activity increased fat intake has similar effects, whereas protein does not [37]. One of the most striking features of fasting is a natriuresis, which continues for about 5 days, when it is followed by sodium retention. Plasma renin activity initially falls during fasting, while aldosterone rises transiently [69]. Studies of more gradual and prolonged weight loss have demonstrated reductions of both renin and aldosterone, which occur independently of changs of sodium intake [74].

Since both caloric restriction and sodium restriction may lower blood pressure, and usually the two go hand in hand, it has been questioned which mechanism is more important in this regard. Fagerberg et al. [21] randomized obese hypertensive men to receive for 10 weeks a diet that was restricted in either calories but not sodium, or one that was restricted in both. Blood pressure fell with the latter, but not the former, suggesting that sodium restriction was the most important component. Plasma norepinephrine showed a greater decrease when both sodium and calories were restricted. Reactivity to infused norepinephrine was increased when calories alone were restricted, but not when both calories and sodium were. These findings led Fagerberg to suggest that although sympathetic nervous activity fell in both cases, increased vascular reactivity may have prevented the blood pressure from falling in the former case.

HEMODYNAMIC CHANGES ASSOCIATED WITH CHANGES IN SODIUM INTAKE

Normotensive Subjects

A number of studies have investigated the hemodynamic effects of changing sodium intake in normal subjects. Abboud [1] and Kirkendall et al. [34] found that going from a low (10 mEq/day) to a high (410 mEq/day) sodium intake did not raise arterial pressure, because there was a decrease of forearm vascular resistance occurring as a result of vasodilation. Similarly, Sullivan and Ratts [70] found that increasing sodium intake from 10 to 200 mEq/day decreased peripheral resistance but raised cardiac output, again with no change of arterial pressure. Finally, Luft et al. [44] found that raising sodium intake from 10 to 300 mEq/day did not increase blood pressure, although there was a modest increase at very high levels of sodium intake (800 to 1500 mEq/day). This was due to an increased cardiac output, but peripheral resistance was again lower.

Several mechanisms may be responsible for these changes. Central venous pressure increases with sodium loading, which would tend to increase cardiac output. The vasodilation might occur as a reflex mediated by stimulation of low-pressure baroreceptors [83]. In addition, the activity of the renin-angiotensin system will be reduced.

Hypertensive Subjects

In contrast to the vasodilator effects of a high sodium intake in normal subjects, Mark et al. [49] found that increasing sodium intake from 10 to 410 mEq/day in subjects with borderline hypertension tended to increase both arterial pressure and forearm vascular resistance. These results were confirmed by Koolen and Van Brummelen [35], who showed that the reflex vasoconstrictor response to lower-body negative pressure (mediated by low-pressure receptors) was enhanced by the high sodium diet in hypertensives, but they also observed a decreased maximal vasodilator capacity (during reactive hyperemia) in sodium-sensitive individuals (i.e., those whose blood pressure varied according to their sodium intake). This finding would suggest that there were structural changes in the arteries occurring with sodium loading, and that the vasoconstriction is not necessarily all mediated neurally.

EFFECTS OF SODIUM INTAKE ON THE SYMPATHETIC NERVOUS SYSTEM

The relationship between sodium intake and sympathetic nervous function is a complex one. A number of studies have indicated that dietary or diuretic-induced sodium depletion can increase plasma catecholamines, which are commonly thought to reflect sympathetic nervous activity [45,76,78]. Conversely, sodium loading has variously been reported to result in a reduction of plasma catecholamines [45], no change [36], or an increase [55]. The latter group reported that the relationship between norepinephrine and sodium intake was U-shaped, with increases of norepinephrine occurring at both extremes of sodium intake. Plasma epinephrine was unaffected by changes of sodium intake.

These apparently conflicting reports on the response to sodium loading may to some extent be attributable to differences in the responses of different subjects. Thus, Koolen and Van Brummelen [35] found that sodium depletion increased plasma norepinephrine in both sodium-sensitive and sodium-resistant hypertensive subjects, but sodium loading produced different effects. Initially, both groups showed a decrease, but after two weeks plasma norepinephrine remained low in the sodium-resistant subjects, but increased to above basal levels in the sodium-sensitive subjects, in whom there was also a significant correlation between the change of blood pressure and of norepinephrine. A temporal component of these relationships was also demonstrated by Volpe [76a], who found that the increased norepinephrine occurring during sodium depletion persisted only for 1 to 2 weeks.

Studies of the effects of sodium depletion on other indices of sympathetic nervous activity have given a very different picture. For example, Ljundqvist [40] found that sodium depletion causes a depletion of norepinephrine from adrenergic nerve terminals in the rat, and Rocchini et al. [63] demonstrated a diminished pressor response to carotid artery occlusion in sodium-depleted dogs. Finally, Takeshita and Ferrario [72] found that sympathetic nerve activity measured directly in the renal nerves of sodium-depleted dogs was diminished in comparison to sodium-replete dogs. Brosnihan et al. [8] reported that sodium depletion causes changes of plasma catecholamines in dogs that are the same as observed in man, namely an increase of norepinephrine without any change of epinephrine. They also found that the concentration of norepinephrine in the cerebrospinal fluid was increased, which they attributed to an increased activity of brain stem noradrenergic neurons. This would be consistent with a decreased central sympathetic outflow, since norepinephrine injected into the brainstem lowers blood pressure [17]. These animal studies would therefore suggest that sodium depletion reduces sympathetic nervous activity.

Human studies of sympathetic responsiveness as a function of sodium intake are few. Ambrosioni et al [2] observed that sodium restriction has relatively little effect on the basal blood pressure in young subjects with borderline hypertension, but the pressor response to stress (dynamic and isometric exercise, and mental arithmetic) was diminished. Similar conclusions were reached by Falkner et al. [22], who found that sodium loading increased the pressor response to mental arithmetic. In contrast, in normal subjects Volpe et al. found that the response to isometric exercise was transiently increased during sodium restriction.

In normotensive subjects, sodium loading increases the pressor sensitivity to infused norepinephrine [59].

If the interpretation of animal studies is correct, why should a decreased level of sympathetic nerve activity during dietary sodium restriction be associated with an increased plasma norepinephrine? A possible explanation is that the increased angiotensin, which also occurs in response to sodium depletion, stimulates the adrenals to release norepinephrine. This effect has been demonstrated experimentally in response to hemorrhage [23]; however, in man, Nicholls et al. [55] did not observe any increase of plasma catecholamines in response to an angiotensin infusion.

At the other end of the spectrum, animal experiments have indicated that sodium loading tends to increase sympathetic activity, and that the sympathetic nervous system plays an important role in mediating experimental models of hypertension that have traditionally been regarded as being sodium-dependent. These include DOCA-salt hypertension [62], one-kidney, one-clip renovascular hypertension [77], and the subtotally nephrectomized rat on a high-salt diet [19]. Gavras [26] has recently proposed the hypothesis that sodium exerts its hypertensive effect by a central effect on adrenergic neurons.

It does not necessarily follow that the interpretation of the animal data that sympathetic activity is diminished by sodium depletion applies to man, because it is conceivable that the assumption of the upright posture necessitates a dual defense mechanism maintaining blood pressure during sodium depletion, and that both the sympathetic nervous system and the renin-angiotensin system are activated.

EFFECTS OF SYMPATHETIC NERVOUS ACTIVITY
ON SODIUM EXCRETION

Activation of the sympathetic nervous system may reduce sodium excretion by its effects both on the renal vasculature and on the renal tubules. Intense stimulation of the renal sympathetic nerves or norepinephrine infusion may reduce renal blood flow and glomerular filtration rate via alpha-adrenergic vasoconstriction [24]. Redistribution of renal blood flow also occurs, with a shunting of blood away from the superficial cortex and toward the medulla, a change that favors sodium reabsorption [57]. There is also a direct effect of sympathetic nervous stimulation on renal tubular sodium reabsorption [18]. Thus, renal denervation produces a natriuresis which is independent of changes of glomerular filtration rate [4].

These effects may be offset by other changes over the long term. Thus, while infusing norepinephrine in man initially causes renal sodium retention, prolonged infusions over several days result in a natriuresis, perhaps as a result of the increased blood pressure, and a progressive decrease in pressor sensitivity [3].

If it is indeed true that increasing sodium intake augments sympathetic nervous activity, which would in turn promote renal sodium retention, there exists the possibility of a positive feedback loop, which could be of relevance during periods of exposure to stress, when there may be both an increased sympathetic activity and an increased salt appetite [16].

EFFECTS OF SODIUM INTAKE ON THE
RENIN-ANGIOTENSIN SYSTEM

The renin-angiotensin-aldosterone system is the principal mechanism by which the effects of sodium depletion are countered. There is a well-documented inverse relationship between sodium intake and plasma renin activity [38], and unlike the apparently transient effects of sodium depletion on plasma catecholamines, renin remains high indefinitely. The renin system acts to maintain homeostasis in two ways: first, by causing an angiotensin-mediated vasoconstriction, and second, by the effects of increased aldosterone secretion to cause sodium retention by the kidney. The physiological importance of angiotensin in maintaining blood pressure during sodium depletion was demonstrated in an experiment by Gavras et al. [27], who showed that saralasin, a competitive angiotensin antagonist, lowered blood pressure in hypertensive patients when they were on a low-sodium diet, but not when on a high-sodium diet.

The vasoconstrictor effects of the increased circulating levels of angiotensin II during sodium depletion may to some extent be offset by the fact that there is down-regulation of the number of vascular angiotensin receptors, which occurs in response to the high plasma angiotensin. Thus, vascular sensitivity to angiotensin may be diminished during sodium depletion, although adrenal sensitivity may be increased [56].

Just as some hypertensive subjects may fail to suppress their plasma catecholamines during sodium loading, so there may be abnormalities in the response of the renin-angiotensin system. Luetscher et al. [43] reported that many hypertensive subjects fail to show the normal suppression of either renin or aldosterone during sodium loading. A similar observation was made by Tuck et al. [75], who reported that more than half of normal renin hypertensive subjects showed a delayed suppression of renin and aldosterone during saline infusion.

In response to sodium depletion, hypertensive subjects who are sodium-sensitive are more likely to have a smaller reactive rise in plasma renin activity [39,67]. Similarly, in patients with refractory hypertension, the blood pressure response to sodium depletion is negatively correlated with the degree of hyperreninemia [28].

EFFECTS OF THE RENIN-ANGIOTENSIN SYSTEM ON SODIUM EXCRETION

In contrast to the transient effects of norepinephrine infusions, angiotensin infusions in normal subjects cause a marked sodium retention, accompanied by an increased pressor sensitivity [3]. After a 3–5-day period, escape occurs with a stabilization of renal sodium excretion. Angiotensin also produces an increased aldosterone secretion, which is the principal mediator of the sodium retention. Aldosterone acts mainly at the level of the distal nephron to decrease sodium excretion and increase the excretion of potassium and hydrogen ions.

Angiotensin also has a direct sodium-retaining effect on the kidney, however. Low-level intrarenal infusion of angiotensin in the dog produces an immediate reduction of sodium and potassium excretion, followed by a gradual rise of arterial pressure [41]. This was not attributable to increased aldosterone secretion, because no kaliuresis was observed. Both glomerular filtration rate and renal plasma flow were decreased, with a rise of filtration fraction, which would be consistent with a preferential action of angiotensin on the efferent arteriole.

In normal subjects, sodium restriction causes a decrased renal blood flow, and sodium loading an increase [80]. These changes are also thought to be mediated by the renin-angiotensin system, and would act in concert with the effects of aldosterone. The increased renal blood flow during sodium loading may help to excrete the sodium load without raising blood pressure.

In patients with hypertension, the acute effects of angiotension are different, and a diuresis results. If, however, the blood pressure is treated, the normal antidiuretic response may be observed [10].

PATHOPHYSIOLOGICAL DETERMINANTS
OF SODIUM SENSITIVITY

Experiments performed in rats have conclusively demonstrated that sodium sensitivity can be genetically determined. The best known example is Dahl's strain of S (sodium-sensitive) and R (sodium-resistant) rats. Although these strains have been studied most extensively to investigate the mechanisms by which sodium can raise blood pressure, it should also be emphasized that the S rats are also more susceptible to other types of hypertension that do not involve excess salt intake, such as Goldblatt renovascular hypertension [15] and psychological stress [25]. The inheritance of sodium sensitivity in these rats is polygenic, and a number of potential mediators have been described, which involve the kidney, adrenal cortex, and nervous system [60].

In recent years, there has been a major effort to identify genetically determined abnormalities of sodium transport across membranes, which might be markers for essential hypertension. Most of these studies have been conducted on membranes taken from red or white cells, although the pathological role of such a defect should be exerted either via the kidneys or vascular smooth muscle. In addition, a variety of transport mechanisms have been studied, and so far no clear picture has emerged. In the words of one recent reviewer of this topic, "We are confronted with a bewildering (and perhaps excessive) array of observations, including many apparently contradictory ones" [6]. Most of these studies have attempted to relate the marker of interest to the presence or absence of hypertension: A more promising approach might be to relate them to the presence or absence of sodium sensitivity. This has recently been attempted by Miller et al. [52], who have reported that haptoglobin typing may be correlated with sodium sensitivity.

The above considerations might imply that sodium sensitivity is one of the heritable factors that predispose individuals to develop hypertension. Thus, Skrabal et al. (1984) found that sodium-sensitive subjects are nearly three times as likely to have a family history of hypertension as sodium-resistant subjects. This, however, was not confirmed by Watt et al. who found no evidence that subjects with a family history of hypertension are more susceptible to dietary sodium than those with a negative family history.

Several potential physiological mediators of sodium sensitivity have been identified. Most prominent among these is the renin-angiotensin system. Dahl S rats have lower renins than R rats [60], and studies in man have shown that the blood-pressure response to sodium restriction is determined by the reactivity of the renin-angiotensin system [12]. Sodium-sensitive subjects have a lower plasma renin activity than sodium-resistant subjects while on a low-sodium diet, and they may also retain more sodium while on a high-sodium diet [33], although this latter finding is controversial [11].

Within the high and normal renin groups of hypertensive patients there may also be considerable variations in the degree of sodium sensitivity. Williams and Hollenberg [80] have suggested that sodium-sensitive patients may be what they term "nonmodulators"—that is, they fail to show the modulation of aldosterone and renal blood flow that normally occur in response to angiotension changes brought about by changing dietary sodium intake. Thus, renal blood flow in the nonmodulators remains relatively constant when dietary sodium in increased, and they also retain more sodium and show an increased blood pressure [61]. These findings are consistent with an earlier study by Brown et al. [9], who reported that sodium-sensitive hypertensive subjects were more likely to retain sodium on a high-salt diet than sodium-resistant subjects. The sodium retention was manifested by changes of total exchangeable sodium, but not of plasma volume.

Myers and Morgan [53] reported that sodium-sensitive subjects were likely to be older, with slightly higher blood pressures and lower creatinine clearances than sodium-resistant subjects. Changes of body weight associated with changes of sodium intake were similar in the two groups, although with sodium loading hematocrit rose in the sodium-sensitive group and fell in the resistant group. These findings led the authors to argue that changes of plasma volume were unlikely to be responsible for mediating the effects on blood pressure.

As discussed above, sodium loading induces vasoconstriction in sodium-sensitive subjects, but not in sodium-resistant ones. A parallel observation is that sodium loading suppresses plasma catecholamines in sodium-resistant individuals, but not in sodium-sensitive ones, which would be consistent with a sodium-induced activation of the sympathetic nervous system in sodium-sensitive individuals [11,35]. Sodium-sensitive subjects also appear to be more sensitive to the pressor effects of infused norepinephrine [67]. Other evidence for a role of the sympathetic nervous system in determining sodium sensitivity comes from the work of Howe et al. [30], who found that denervation of the baroreceptors of normotensive Wistar-Kyoto rats made them more sodium sensitive.

Another mechanism that has been proposed to explain sodium sensitivity is that there is a circulating natriuretic hormone whose main action would be to inhibit sodium transport across the renal tubules, perhaps by inhibiting NA-K ATPase, but that might also act on vascular smooth muscle to increase peripheral resistance [46]. Although claims have been made for the isolation of such a substance, its existence and importance remain controversial [14].

REFERENCES

1. Abboud FM (1984): Effects of sodium, angiotensin, and steroids on vascular reactivity in man. Fed Proc 33:143–149.

2. Ambrosioni E, Costa FV, Borghi C, Montebugnoli L, Giordani MF, Magnami B (1982): Effects of moderate salt restriction on intralymphocytic sodium and pressor response to stress in borderline hypertension. Hypertension 4:789–794.

3. Ames RP, Borkowski AJ, Sicinski AM, Laragh JH (1965): Prolonged infusions of angiotensin II and norepinephrine and blood pressure, electrolyte balance, and aldosterone and cortisol secretion in normal man and in cirrhosis with ascites. J Clin Invest 44: 1171–1186.

4. Bello-Reuss E, Trevino DL, Gottschalk CW (1976): Effect of renal sympathetic nerve stimulation on proximal water and sodium reabsorption. J Clin Invest 57:1104–1107.

5. Berglund G, Larson B, Andersson O, Larsson O, Svärdsudd K, Bjorntorp P, Wilhelmsen L (1976): Body composition and glucose metabolism in hypertensive middle-aged males. Acta Med Scand 200:163–169.

6. Blaustein MP (1984) Sodium transport and hypertension. Where are we going? Hypertension 6:445–453.

7. Boehringer K, Beretta-Piccoli C, Weidmann P, Meier A, Ziegler W (1982): Pressor factors and cardiovascular pressor responsiveness in lean and overweight normal or hypertensive subjects. Hypertension 4:697–702.

8. Brosnihan KB, Szilagyi JE, Ferrario CM (1981): Effect of chornic sodium depletion or cerebrospinal fluid and plasma catecholamines. Hypertension 3:233–239.

9. Brown WJ, Brown FK, Krisham I (1971): Exchangeable sodium and blood volume in normotensive and hypertensive humans on high and low sodium intake. Circulation 43: 508–519.

10. Brown JJ, Peart WS (1962): The effect of angiotensin on urine flow and electrolyte excretion in hypertensive patients. Clin Sci 22:1–17.

11. Campese VM (1982): Salt and neurogenic variables in essential hypertension. In Iwai J. Igako-Shoin (ed): Salt and Hypertension. New York/Tokyo pp 259–274.

12. Cappuccio FP, Markandu ND, Sagnella GA, MacGregor GA (1985): Sodium restriction lowers high blood pressure through a decreased response of the renin system-direct evidence using saralasin. J Hypertension 3:234–247.

13. Chiang VN, Perlman LV, Epstein FH (1969): Overweight and hypertension: A review. Circ. 39: 403-410.

14. Cloix JFC, Crabos M, Meyer P (1986): Recent progress on an endogenous digitalis-like factor in hypertension. J Clin Hypertension 2:93–100.

15. Dahl LK, Heine M, Tassinari L (1963): Effects of chronic excess salt ingestion. Role of genetic factors in both DOCA-salt and renal hypertension. J Exp Med 118:605–617.

16. Denton DA, Coghlan JP, Fei DT, McKinley M, Nelson J, Scoggins B, Tarjan E, Tregear GW, Tresham JJ, Weisinger R (1984): Stress, ACTH, salt intake and high blood pressure. Clin Exp Hyper A5:403–415.

17. DeJong W (1974): Noradrenaline: central inhibitory control of pressure and heart rate. Eur J Pharmacol 29:179–181.

18. DiBona GF (1977): Neurogenic regulation of renal tubular sodium reabsorption. Amer J Physiol 233:F73–81.

19. DePette D, Waeber B, Volicer L, Chao P, Gavras I, Gavras H, Brunner H (1983): Salt-induced hypertension in chronic renal failure: Evidence for a neurogenic mechanism. Life Sci 32:733–740, 1983.

20. Divitis D, Fazio S, Petitto M, Maddenalena G, Contaldo F, Mancini M (1981): Obesity and cardiac function. Circ 64:477–482.
21. Fagerberg B, Andersson OK, Persson B, Hedner T (1985): Reactivity to norepinephrine and effect of sodium on blood pressure during weight loss. Hypertension 7:586–592.
22. Falkner B, Onesti G, Angelakos E (1981): Effect of salt loading on the cardiovascular response to stress in adolescents. Hypertension 3 (suppl. II):195–199.
23. Feuerstein G, Boonyaviroj P, Gutman Y (1977): Renin-angiotensin mediation of adrenal catecholamine secretion induced by hemorrhage. Eur J Pharmacol 44:131–142.
24. Fink ED, Brody MJ (1978): Continuous measurement of renal blood flow changes to renal nerve stimulation and intra-arterial drug administration in the rat. Amer J Physiol 234: H219–222.
25. Friedman R, Iwai J (1976): Genetic predisposition and stress-induced hypertension. Science 193:161–162.
26. Gavras H (1986): How does salt raise blood pressure? A hypothesis. Hypertension 8: 83–86.
27. Gavras H, Ribiero AB, Gavras I, Brunner HR (1976): Reciprocal relation between renin dependency and sodium dependency in essential hypertension. New Engl J Med 295: 1278–1283.
28. Gavras H, Waeber B, Kershaw GR, Liang CS, Textor SC, Brunner HR, Tifft CB, Gavras IH (1981): Role of reactive hyperreninemia in blood pressure changes induced by sodium depletion in patients with refractory hypertension. Hypertension 3:441–447.
29. Halliday D, Hesp R, Stalley SF, Warwick P, Altman DG, Garrow JS (1979): Resting metabolic rate, weight, surface area, and body composition in obese women. Int J Obesity 3:1–6.
30. Howe PR, Rogers PF, Minson JB (1985): Influence of dietary sodium on blood pressure in baroreceptor-denervated rats. J Hypertension 3:457–460.
31. Jung RT, Shetty PS, Barrand M, Callingham BA, James WPT (1979): Role of catecholamines in hypotensive response to dieting. Brit Med J 1:12–13.
32. Kaltman AJ, Golding RM (1976): Role of circulatory congestion in the cardiorespiratory failure of obesity. Amer J Med 60:645–653.
33. Kawaski T, Delea CS, Barttler FC, Smith H (1978): The effect of high-sodium and low-sodium intakes on blood pressure and other related variables in human subjects with idiopathic hypertension. Amer J Med 64:193–198.
34. Kirkendall WM, Connor WE, Abboud FM, Rustogi SP, Anderson TA, Fry M (1976): The effect of dietary sodium chloride on blood pressure, body fluids, electrolytes, renal function, and serum lipids of normotensive man. J Lab Clin Med 87:418–434.
35. Koolen MI, Van Brummelen P (1984): Adrenergic activity and peripheral hemodynamics in relation to sodium sensitivity in patients with essential hypertension. Hypertension 6:820–825.
36. Lake CR, Ziegler MG (1977): Effect of acute volume alterations on norepinephrine and dopamine-β-hydroxylase in normotensive and hypertensive subjects. Circ 57:774–777.
37. Landsberg L, Young JB (1986): Caloric intake and sympathetic nervous system activity. Implications for blood pressure regulation and thermogenesis. J Clin Hypertension 2: 166–171.
38. Laragh JH (1973): Vasoconstriction-volume analysis for understanding and treating hypertension. The use of renin and aldosterone profiles. Am J Med 55:261–274.
39. Laragh JH, Pecker MS (1983): Dietary sodium and essential hypertension: Some myths, hopes, and truths. Ann Int Med 98:735–743.
40. Ljundqvist A (1975): The effect of angiotension infusion, sodium loading, and sodium

restriction on the renal and cardiac adrenergic nerves. Acta Path Microbiol Scand 83: 661–668.

41. Lohmeier TE, Cowley AW (1979): Hypertensive and renal effects of chronic low level intrarenal angiotensin infusion in the dog. Circ Res 44:154–160.

42. Lucas CP, Estigarribia JA, Darga LL, Reaven GM (1985): Insulin and blood pressure in obesity. Hypertension 7:702–706.

43. Luetscher JA, Beckerhoff R, Dowdy AJ, Wilkinson R (1972): Incomplete suppression of aldosterone secretion and plasma concentration in hypertensive patients on high sodium intake. In Genest J, Koiw E (eds): "Hypertension '72." Berlin: Springer, pp 286–292.

44. Luft FC, Rankin LI, Bloch R, Weyman AE, Willis LR, Murray RH, Brimm CE, Weinberger MH (1979a): Cardiovascular and humoral responses to extremes of sodium intake in normal black and white men. Circulation 60:697–706.

45. Luft FC, Rankin LI, Henry DP, Bloch R, Grim CE, Weyman AE, Murray RC, Weinberger MH (1979b): Plasma and urinary norepinephrine values at extremes of sodium intake in normal man. Hypertension 1:261–266.

46. MacGregor GA (1983): Sodium and potassium intake and blood pressure. Hypertension 5 (suppl. III):79–84.

47. MacMahon SW, MacDonald GJ, Bernstein L, Andrews G, Blacket RB (1985): Comparison of weight reduction with metoprolol in treatment of hypertension of young overweight patients. Lancet 2:1233–1236.

48. Mancini M, Strazzullo P (1986): Energy balance and blood-pressure regulation. Update and future perspectives. J Clin Hypertension 2:148–153.

49. Mark AL, Lawton WJ, Abboud FM, Fitz AE, Connor WE, Heistad DD (1975): Effects of high and low sodium intake on arterial pressure and forearm vascular resistance in borderline hypertension: A preliminary report. Circ Res 36:I194–198.

50. Messerli FH (1984): Obesity in hypertension: How innocent a bystander? Amer J Med 77:1077–1082.

51. Messerli FH, Christie B, deCarvalho JGR, Aristiono GG, Suarez DGH, Dreslinski GR, Frohlich ED (1981): Obesity and essential hypertension: hemodynamics, intravascular volume, sodium excretion, and plasma renin activity. Arch Int Med 141:81–85.

52. Miller JZ, Weinberger NH, Fineberg NS, Grim CE (1986): Haptoglobin: A genetic marker for sodium sensitivity of blood pressure? Circ. 74, II-329 (abstract).

53. Myers JB, Morgan TO (1983): Alterations in renal function and haematocrit in normal people who have a rise of blood pressure with extra sodium. New Z Med J 96:895–897.

54. Nicholls MG, Espiner EA, Miles KE, Swiefler AJ, Julius S (1981): Evidence against an interaction of angiotensin II with the sympathetic nervous system in man. Clin Endocrinol 15:423–430.

55. Nicholls MG, Kiowski W, Zweifler AJ, Julius S, Schork MA, Greenhouse J (1980): Plasma norepinephrine variations with dietary sodium intake. Hypertension 2:29–32.

56. Olsen ME, Meydrech EF (1985): Physiological responses to angiotensin II infusion during chronic angiotensin converting enzyme inhibition in dogs on normal, low and high sodium intake. J Hypertension 3:517–525.

57. Pomeranz BH, Birtch AG, Barger AC (1968): Neural control of intrarenal blood flow. Amer J Physiol 215:1067–1081.

58. Raison J, Archrinastos A, Asmar R, Simon A, Safar M (1986): Extracellular and interstitial fluid volume in obesity with and without associated systemic hypertension. Amer J Cardiol 57:223–226.

59. Rankin LI, Luft FC, Henry DP, Gibbs PS, Weinberger MH (1981): Sodium intake alters the effects of norepinephrine on blood pressure. Hypertension 3:650–656.

60. Rapp JP (1982): Dahl salt-susceptible and salt-resistant rats. Hypertension 4:753–756.
61. Redgrave JE, Rabinowe SL, Hollenberg NK, Williams GH (1985): Correction of abnormal renal blood flow response to angiotensin II by converting enzyme inhibition in essential hypertensives. J Clin Invest 75:1285–1290.
62. Reid JL, Zivin JA, Kopin IJ (1975): Central and peripheral adrenergic mechanisms in the development of deoxycorticosterone-saline hypertension in rats. Circ Res 37:569–579.
63. Rocchini AP, Cant JR, Barger AC (1977): Carotid sinus reflex in dogs with low- to high-sodium intake. Amer J Physiol 233:H196–202.
64. Rowe JW, Young JB, Minaker KL, Steven AL, Pallotta J, Landsberg L (1981): Effects of insulin and glucose infusion in sympathetic nervous activity in normal man. Diabetes 30:219–225.
65. Schwartz JH, Young JB, Landsberg L (1983): Effect of dietary fat on sympathetic nervous system activity in the rat. J Clin Invest 72:361–370.
66. Sims EAH (1982): Mechanisms of hypertension in the overweight. Hypertension 4 (suppl III):43–49.
67. Skrabal F, Herholz H, Neumayr M, Hamberger L, Ledochowski M, Sporer H, Hörtnagl H, Schwarz S, and Schömitzer D (1984): Salt sensitivity in human is linked to enhanced sympathetic responsiveness and to enhanced proximal tubular reabsorption. Hypertension 6:152–158.
68. Sowers JR, Whitfield LA, Beck FJW, Cataina TA, Tuck ML, Domfeld L, Maxwell M (1982): Role of enhanced sympathetic nervous system activity and reduced Na, K dependent adenosine triphosphatase activity in maintenance of elevated blood pressure in obesity: Effects of weight loss. Clin Sc 63 (suppl 8):121S–124S.
69. Spark RF, Arky RA, Boutler PR, Saudek CD, O'Brian JT (1975): Renin, aldosterone and glucagon in the natriuresis of fasting. New Engl J Med 292:1335–1340.
70. Sullivan JM, Ratts TE (1983): Hemodynamic mechanisms of adaptation to chronic high sodium intake in normal humans. Hypertension 5:814–820.
71. Sullivan JM, Ratts TE, Taylor JC, Krasu DH, Barton BR, Patrick DR, Reed SW (1980): Hemodynamic effects of dietary sodium in man. Hypertension 2:506–514.
72. Takeshita S, Ferrario CM (1982): Altered neural control of cardiovascular function in sodium-depleted dogs. Hypertension 4 (suppl II):175–182.
73. Takeshita A, Imaizumi T, Ashihara T, Nakamura M (1982): Characteristics of responses to salt loading and deprivation in hypertensive subjects. Circ Res 51:457–464.
74. Tuck ML, Sowers J, Dornfeld K, Kledzik G, Maxwell M (1981): The effect of weight reduction on blood pressure, plasma renin activity, and plasma aldosterone levels in obese patients. New Engl J Med 304:930–933.
75. Tuck ML, Williams GH, Dluhy RG, Greenfield M, Moore TJ (1976): A delayed suppression of the renin-aldosterone axis following saline infusion in human hypertension. Circ Res 39:711–717.
76. Vitiello MV, Prinz PN, Halter JB (1983): Sodium-restricted diet increases nighttime plasma norepinephrine and impairs sleep patterns in man. J Clin Endocrinol Metab 50:553–556.
76a. Volpe M, Muller FB, Trimarco B. Transient enhancement of sympathetic nervous system activity by long-term restriction of sodium intake. Circulation 72, 47–52–, 1985.
77. Waeber B, Gavras H, Gavras I, et al. (1982): Evidence for a sodium-induced activation of central mechanisms in one-kidney, one-clip renal hypertension. J Pharmacol Exp Ther 233:510–515.
78. Warren SE, Vieweg WVR, O'Connor DT (1980): Sympathetic nervous system activity during sodium restriction in essential hypertension. Clin Cardiol 3:348–351.
79. Watt GCM, Goy CJW, Hart JT (1986): Dietary sodium and blood pressure in young people

with and without familial predisposition to high blood pressure. J Clin Hypertension 2:141–147.

80. Williams GH, Hollenberg NK (1985): Non-modulating essential hypertension: A subset particularly responsive to converting enzyme inhibitors. J Hypertension 3 (suppl 2):S81–S87.

81. Young JB, Landsberg L (1977a): Stimulation of the sympathetic nervous system during sucrose feeding. Nature 269:615–617.

82. Young JB, Landsberg L (1977b): Suppression of sympathetic nervous system during fasting. Science 196:1473–1475.

83. Zoller RP, Mark AL, Abboud FM, Schmid PG, Heistad DD (1972): The role of low pressure baroreceptors in reflex vasoconstrictor responses in man. J Clin Invest 51:2967–2972.

Nutritional Factors in Hypertension
© *1990 Alan R. Liss, Inc., pages 17–34*

2 | # Epidemiology of Nutrition and Hypertension

Sylvia Wassertheil-Smoller, Ph.D.
Bernard Lamport, M.D.

INTRODUCTION

Epidemiology as a discipline often yields the first clues concerning the etiology of certain diseases. The examination of rates, one of the principal statistics in epidemiology, and the drawing of inferences from those rates, may suggest interventional strategies that can then be tested through clinical trials. Prevalence rates of hypertension vary widely among different populations. Such variability leads one to speculate about the concomitant differences in environmental or life-style conditions that exist within those societies and to compare and contrast such factors in societies where the prevalence of hypertension is low with those where the prevalence is high. Diet is one such factor that has generated increasing attention.

METHODOLOGICAL ISSUES

First, it is important to consider some of the methodological issues involved in drawing inferences about the relationship of diet and disease. The first issue concerns inferences drawn from the intersociety comparisons. Intersociety descriptors of diet generally rest on food-consumption data, and the problem with inferences made from such data is that coincident with variations in food consumption are differences in other life-style and environmental patterns. For example, societies that have higher intakes of pro-

From the Department of Epidemiology and Social Medicine, Albert Einstein College of Medicine, 1300 Morris Park Avenue, Bronx, NY 10461.

cessed foods are also societies that are more industrialized than those with lower usage, and thus to tease out which of the factors are more important in their relation to hypertension becomes very difficult from such data.

The second issue concerns intrasociety comparisons. Often, it is not possible to show a relationship between diet and hypertension within a particular society because of the homogeneity of the population with regard to intake of a particular nutrient. Within a homogeneous population, it may be that the variation of a dietary factor within the same individual from day to day may be as large or larger than the variation of that factor among individuals. For nutrients of high intraindividual variability, it is difficult to estimate accurately the true "habitual" intake for each individual.

Third, assessment of dietary intake is difficult and a variety of methods are used, each of which has certain limitations. For example, assessing dietary intake through food-frequency diet histories where the individuals estimate how often they eat a particular food may have the advantage of getting information about past intake. This is important because any etiological factor would have to exert its influence over a long period of time prior to the development of hypertension. There is considerable literature on the use of retrospective estimates of dietary intake [1–4], and for the most part there is agreement that diet history through food-frequency method is reliable when no known changes occur in the diet of the respondent [2]. However, it has also been found that current diet influences estimates of past diet [3]. People are more likely to recall having eaten something that they are currently eating. On the positive side, however, studies have found high correlations between repeat diet histories at six-month and two-year intervals [5,6] for fat, protein, and calories.

Another way of assessing dietary intake is through a 24-hour recall where the patient, with the help of a nutritionist, recalls what he ate in the past 24 hours. This is probably a more accurate way of assessing intake than the food-frequency questionnaires and may be adequate for characterizing group intake, but it is not adequate for characterizing the habitual intake of individuals. Food records where the individual keeps a diary of his intake over a period of one or more days eliminates the problem of remembering what has been eaten, since intake is recorded as foods are consumed, but may have limitations due to compliance, since it may be somewhat cumbersome to keep such records. However, it is generally considered to be the more accurate way of estimating intake.

While it is widely recognized that fewer number of days of recorded intake are required to characterize group averages for intergroup comparisons, in order to estimate an individual's usual intake a longer period of records is necessary [7–9]. Sempos [8] has stated that it would require two to thirty days of food records, depending on the nutrient of interest. This is a reflection of the intraindividual variability of certain nutrients. The problem here is to estimate the true correlation between nutrient intake and the physiological characteristic of interest—in this case, blood pressure. The efficiency of such estimation is dependent on R^2x, which is the ratio of intra- to interindividual variance for the nutrient in question, and R^2y, which is the ratio of intra- to interindividual variance for the physiological marker—i.e., blood pressure. We have calculated the number of days of food records required to establish the association between a given nutrient and blood pressure based on the methodology presented by Liu [7]. Our data were obtained from the multicenter Trial of Antihypertensive Interventions and Management (TAIM). The TAIM study is intended to determine an optimal combination of drug and diet therapy for mild hypertension with respect to control of blood pressure, life satisfaction variables, and minimization of side effects. We estimated the ratio of intraindividual to interindividual variance calculated by analysis of variance components based on 867 individuals, each of whom had a 3-day food record collected at the baseline of the TAIM study. Assuming that there is no intraindividual variation in blood pressure (not a very reasonable assumption, but used here for illustrative purposes), Table 1 below indicates the number of food records necessary to estimate the true correlation coefficient between the nutrient and blood pressure with 90% efficiency. As can be seen, the number of food records required ranges from 4 to 7 days. Sodium which has large intraindividual variation requires 7 days, while calories require 4 days. These estimates are conservative, since in fact the intraindividual variation in the measurement of blood pressure itself would increase the number of days required.

Clearly, collecting that many days of food records and analyzing them is costly, and thus one of our major surveys of food consumption in the United States, the National Health and Nutrition Examination Survey (NHANES), which employs large national samples statistically drawn to represent the United States population, uses the 24-hour dietary recall as the primary means of estimating dietary intake.

Another methodological difficulty has to do with separating out the spe-

TABLE 1. Number of Days of Food Recording Required to Estimate Different Nutrients

	Number of Days required to estimate correlation with 90% efficiency*
Calories	4
Sodium	7
Potassium	4
Calcium	4

*Assuming no intraindividual variability in blood pressure.

cific nutrient components that are closely related to one another and that are responsible for associations with blood pressure either singly or in combination with each other. This issue is discussed by Reed [10] in his analysis of data from a cohort of Japanese men in Hawaii. He pointed out that the data indicate that several dietary factors are inversely related to blood pressure levels independently of other risk factors, such as age, body mass, and alcohol intake. However, the high degree of intercorrelation (multicolinearity) among these dietary factors indicates that the independent role of any specific nutrient cannot be conclusively separated from the possible effects of other nutrients.

A further methodological consideration is whether the data are cross-sectional or longitudinal. Cross-sectional surveys measure the nutrient intake and blood pressure at the same point in time and thus may provide evidence of association but not evidence of causality. Longitudinal surveys obtain estimates of nutrient intake at a certain point in time and follow the same group of individuals into the future to determine the change in blood pressure or the development of hypertension, and thus constitute stronger evidence of etiological relationships. Data from both kinds of surveys will be discussed in the following section.

SODIUM AND CALCIUM: CROSS-SECTIONAL STUDIES

The principal source of cross-sectional data in the United States to examine the relationship of diet to nutritional status comes from the NHANES surveys on food consumption, based on a probability sampling of the United States population 1 to 74 years of age. The first such survey, NHANES-I, was conducted from 1971 to 1974, and the second such survey, NHANES-II, was conducted from 1976 to 1980. These surveys employ the 24-hour recall to obtain information on nutrient intake.

The HANES data have shown conflicting associations between several different nutrients and blood pressure. Figure 1 indicates the degree to which normotensive individuals in the HANES sample consumed an excess of certain nutrients when compared to hypertensive individuals. For example, normotensives consumed 16% more calories than hypertensives. In this analysis of the HANES-I data by McCarron [11–13], normotensives consumed more protein, fat, carbohydrates, calcium, phosphorus, sodium, potassium, vitamin A, cholesterol, vitamin C, and linoleic acid. McCarron concludes that reduced consumption of calcium and potassium is the primary nutritional marker of hypertension, along with reductions in vitamins A and C. In this analysis, diets low in sodium were associated with higher blood pressures, while high-sodium diets were associated with lower blood pressures. Such a conclusion runs counter to the prevailing belief that high sodium is a precursor of hypertension.

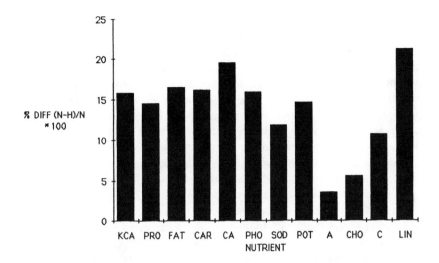

**Fig. 1.   Differences between normotensives and hypertensives in nutrient consumption.
% difference (y coordinate) =**

$$\frac{\text{average consumed by normotensives-average consumed by hypertensives}}{\text{average consumed by normotensives}} \times 100.$$

**KCA, K calories; PRO, protein; FAT, fat; CAR, carbohydrates; CA, calcium; PHO,
phosphorus; SOD, sodium; POT, potassium; A, vitamin A; CHO, cholesterol; C, vitamin
C; LIN, linoleic acid.**

In another analysis of the same data, but using multivariate statistical
techniques rather than direct adjustment, Gruchow and his coinvestigators
[14] found that alcohol and sodium intake and phosphorus were *directly*
related to high blood pressure among U.S. adults, while potassium was
inversely related. Their analysis indicated that calcium intake was significantly related to systolic blood pressure only among nonwhite men and was
not a significant predictor of systolic pressure overall. The most important
point these investigators make is that age, race, and obesity are such strong
determinants of hypertension that current nutrient intakes by comparison are
relatively less important.

There is a continuing debate on whether calcium or sodium is more important in the pathogenesis of essential hypertension. In his review article,
McCarron [15] makes a case for calcium, while MacGregor [16] makes an
equally convincing case for sodium. As a young man responded when he was
asked if he preferred the music of Bach or Beethoven, "Why do I have to
choose?" So it is not necessary to be a partisan of sodium or calcium; neither

or both may be related to hypertension. Sodium intake is the area that has received perhaps the most attention, since early observations by Dahl [17] suggested a relationship to blood pressure, and so the following section presents evidence with regard to sodium and hypertension.

Early intersocietal observations suggested that societies with high intakes of dietary sodium, as measured by urinary sodium excretion, had higher prevalence of hypertension compared to societies with lower sodium intakes. However, there is likely to be some confounding between other factors that impact both on life-style and sodium intake, and hence blood pressure. For example, northern Japan, which has the highest intake of urinary sodium, an average of 425 mEq per person per day, also has among the highest prevalence rates of hypertension (over 40%), while Alaskan Eskimos and people in the New Guinea highlands who show the lowest urinary sodium excretion, 50 mEq or less, have virtually no hypertension [18]. Clearly, these societies differ in ways other than sodium intake.

The intrasocietal studies of sodium and hypertension are complicated, as mentioned before, by the large day-to-day variation of sodium intake by the same individual and by the relatively narrow ranges of intake within the same society. Additionally, when assessing sodium intake by dietary records or recall, it is difficult to get accurate data. The most recent and largest cross-sectional study that provides data on intersocietal as well as intrasocietal cross-sectional relationships between nutrients and hypertension is Intersalt [19]. This was an international study of 10,079 men and women aged 20 to 59 in 52 centers from 32 countries, relating electrolyte excretion to blood pressure and controlling for the confounding variables of body mass and alcohol consumption. Intersalt found in the intrasocietal analyses that, after adjustment for age, sex, body mass index, alcohol consumption, and potassium excretion, and pooling data from the centers, the relation of sodium to systolic blood pressure, but not to diastolic, was significant.

Analyses across centers (intersocietal) indicated that when 4 of the 52 centers that had extremely low sodium excretion were removed from the analyses, neither the prevalence of hypertension nor the median blood pressure was related to sodium excretion. In these four centers with low sodium excretion, the median blood pressures were low and the slopes of blood pressure with age were negative or very small, while in the other centers blood pressure levels were higher in successively higher age groups. Such findings might suggest that lowered sodium intake could prevent the rise of blood pressure with age that is commonly found in industrialized societies. On the other hand, however, it may be likely that there is some threshold effect such that extremely low sodium-intake levels are required before blood pressure is affected. It is not likely that such extremely low levels of intake can be achieved in Western societies. It is estimated that about one-third of sodium intake comes from natural food sources, one-third from processed foods, and one-third as added salt. Thus, while there was some indication of a relationship between sodium and blood pressure, it would be a very weak association at best. In another cross-sectional study, among 7,354 Scots men and women aged 40 to 59, the correlations found between sodium excretion and blood pressure were also very weak [20]. It is not likely that more cross-sectional studies of sodium and blood pressure will yield more conclusive results.

Cross-sectional studies of calcium also yield conflicting interpretations. Sempos [21] compared the HANES-I and HANES-II surveys with regard to dietary calcium. These analyses do not show an association between low calcium intake and blood pressure, nor do they support the hypothesis that low calcium intakes by blacks can explain blood pressure differences between blacks and whites. In contrast to the contradictory evidence about dietary calcium and its relation to blood pressure, there appears to be a highly consistent relationship between total calcium (including supplements) and blood pressure.

Schramm et al. [22], in a cross-sectional study, looked at the relationship between blood pressure and current calcium intake in 199 white postmenopausal women (46 to 66 years old) with no history of hypertension. They found no significant correlation between calcium intake and blood pressure even after controlling for other known risk factors for hypertension. One caveat is that since it is known that calcium absorption declines with age, older persons may require much higher doses of calcium to produce an effect on blood pressure.

Kok et al. [23] report on a study of civil servants and their spouses in Amsterdam who were aged 40 to 65 in 1953–1954. This is a cross-sectional study involving 1,247 men and 1,047 women. Dietary data were assessed by one-week food-frequency recalls. It was found that dietary calcium showed a negative association with systolic blood pressure that remained significant in males and females after controlling for confounders. Associations with sodium and potassium, although they were significant inversely in the univariate analyses, were made nonsignificant after controlling for age. In multivariate analyses in females, however, dietary calcium was the only micronutrient that contributed significantly to diastolic blood pressure. These investigators state they cannot provide support for any strong association between calcium and hypertension.

Kaplan and Meese [24] review the evidence on calcium and conclude that there is little support for the basic premise of the calcium-deficiency hypothesis with regard to hypertension, but that this hypothesis deserves further exploration.

LONGITUDINAL STUDIES—MULTIPLE NUTRIENTS

Prospective follow-up studies can theoretically provide stronger evidence of etiological associations between diet and hypertension, though they are subject to the methodological difficulties of assessing intake accurately, maintaining follow-up, and having to analyze dietary variables with high intercorrelations.

The Zutphen study was a longitudinal investigation of the relations between diet and other risk factors and chronic diseases among middle-aged men, carried out in the town of Zutphen in the Netherlands. This is part of the Seven Countries Study, under the direction of Keyes [25]. The Seven Countries Study is concerned with 15 cohorts comprising 11,579 men aged 40 to 59 years and healthy at entry. The Zutphen study was a prospective investigation that started in 1960 and followed participants through 1970; 794 men were examined in 1960 and 498 reexamined in 1970. The method of estimating dietary intake was through dietary history of usual consumption 6 to 12 months prior to the interview. Kromhaut et al. [26] found that potassium was inversely related to systolic blood pressure. Calcium was inversely related to both systolic and diastolic blood pressure, after adjustment for the other nutrients and for caloric intake as well as body-mass index and age. Changes in these nutrients did not produce significant changes in blood pressure, except for alcohol, where, after adjustment, changes in alcohol intake were directly related to change in blood pressure. Sodium intake was not assessed.

The Honolulu Heart Program is a prospective study of coronary heart disease and stroke in a cohort of Japanese men born between 1900 and 1919 and living in Oahu in 1965. Joffers et al. [27] report on an analysis relating nutrient intake to these endpoints in this elderly free-living population. Dietary data were obtained by a 24-hour recall for 615 men. A major finding of the study was that magnesium, both from foods and from supplements, was inversely related to systolic and diastolic blood pressure. It should be pointed out that magnesium from foods and magnesium from supplements were not correlated with each other, but each separately had an inverse relationship to blood pressure. Magnesium, calcium, phosphorus, potassium, fiber, vegetable protein, starch, vitamin C, and vitamin D intake were significant variables that showed inverse associations with blood pressure in univariate and multivariate analyses, with magnesium having the strongest association. All of this indicates that foods such as vegetables, fruits, whole grains, and low-fat dairy items that are major sources of these nutrients may be protective against hypertension. In this study, sodium from food had no association with blood pressure when adjusted for age and body-mass index.

ALCOHOL

Alcohol consumption has been suggested as being directly related to high blood pressure in several studies [28–43], and there is increasing interest in the potential of alcohol reduction for prevention of hypertension.

In a report by Klatsky et al. [38] of 87,000 ambulatory adult subscribers to the Kaiser Permanente medical care program, the investigators found in their cross-sectional study that: 1) regular use of three or more drinks a day is associated with an increased risk of hypertension, independent of confounders, 2) that regular use of less than two drinks a day does not carry such a risk, and 3) that the apparent blood pressure/alcohol relation does not continue beyond six to eight drinks a day in whites or three to five drinks a day in blacks. These relations held for each level of adiposity.

Other cross-sectional studies have also indicated a strong relationship. A positive association between hypertension and alcoholism was found in a study of 6,494 black persons [39], with black alcoholic subjects having a 20% greater chance of having hypertension than control subjects. The Lipid Research Clinics Prevalence Study [40] investigates the relationship between alcohol consumption and blood pressure in 2,482 men and 2,301 women older than 20 years in nine North American populations. Analyses revealed that men and women with the highest level of alcohol consumption ($\geq$30 ml alcohol per day) had the highest blood pressure. It was also found that men over 35 years consuming high doses of alcohol were 1.5 to 2 times more likely to be hypertensive than nondrinkers. The relationship of both systolic and diastolic blood pressure to alcohol consumption was independent of the confounding factors of age, obesity, smoking, regular exercise, education, and gonadal hormones used in women. Regression coefficients showed that, on the average, a 30-ml intake of alcohol per day is associated with a 2- to 6-mmHg higher systolic blood pressure than that in a nondrinker. The Intersalt Study, described previously, also showed a strong significant independent relationship between heavy alcohol use and blood pressure.

A significant positive relationship was found between alcohol intake and blood pressure for men 40 to 69 years old in urban (492 men) and rural (395 men) areas in Japan [41]. The relationship between alcohol and blood pressure was found to be continuous, without threshold, showing an effect of even moderate consumption (22–55 g/day) of alcohol. This is in contrast to some studies that have suggested a U-type relationship, with people consuming low amounts of alcohol faring worse than those consuming moderate amounts.

In a recent report of a cross-sectional study from Michigan of 2,627 individuals, heavier alcohol intakes were associated with increased systolic and diastolic blood pressure and with the prevalence of hypertension [42].

However, attributable risk calculations indicated that no more than 8.5% of instances of elevated blood pressure could be attributed to alcohol intake exceeding one drink a day (four-ounce glass of wine, 12-ounce bottle of beer, or 1.5 ounce of liquor). Potter and Beevers [43] demonstrated, in a small experimental in-hospital study of 16 hypertensive men, that alcohol consumption causes a rise in blood pressure and alcohol withdrawal causes a fall in blood pressure in moderate-drinking (80 g of alcohol daily) hypertensives.

It has been suggested that in general the systolic blood pressure is more sensitive to the influence of alcohol than diastolic blood pressure.

POTASSIUM

An inverse relationship between potassium intake and blood pressure has been suggested by Langford [44] and others. Populations such as the Japanese and Koreans, who have a high salt intake and a low potassium intake, have high prevalence of hypertension and high frequency of stroke. In America, blacks have a substantially lower intake of potassium than whites. In our Dietary Intervention Study of Hypertension (DISH) [45], a clinical trial to determine if drug-treated hypertensives could be withdrawn from medication and have their blood pressure brought under control through dietary modification, we found that black males on the average had a 24-hour urinary potassium excretion of 45 mEq, compared to 82 mEq for white males [46]. The dietary intake estimates were similar. Part of this difference may have been due to the lower reported caloric intake in this sample—1,323 calories for black men vs. 2,240 for white men. However, this is not likely to be a major factor, since the correlation between calories and potassium was only .30 and for women, blacks had both a higher caloric intake and lower potassium than white women (Fig. 2). In our current study of combinations of drugs and diet, the Trial of Antihypertensive Intervention and Management (TAIM), a similar relationship is obtained with blacks having an average dietary intake of 79 mEq compared to whites with intake of 60 mEq (unpublished data).

It is difficult, however, to establish whether sodium intake, potassium intake, or the sodium/potassium ratio is the most important factor. Intersalt reported that, cross-sectionally, the relation of potassium excretion to blood pressure in individual subjects was inverse but weak, and that there was no consistent association across centers. The relation of the sodium/potassium ratio followed a pattern similar to that of sodium. Recently, a prospective study was reported by Khaw and Barrett-Connor on dietary potassium and stroke associated mortality [47]. This was a study of 859 men and women aged 50 to 79, a population-based cohort in southern California (356 men, 503 women without any history of heart attack, heart failure, or stroke at baseline). Dietary intake was measured by 24-hour recall. The dependent

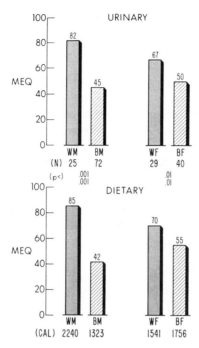

Fig. 2. Potassium intake and urinary excretion by race and sex based on the DISH study. p values refer to comparison between blacks and whites within each sex. Upper p value refers to urinary excretion; lower p value refers to dietary intake. WM, white males; BM, black males; WF, white females; BF, black females; MEQ, milliequivalents; N, number; CAL, calories.

variable was 12-year stroke mortality adjusted for age. The nutrients examined were calories, proteins, saturated and polyunsaturated fat, alcohol, potassium, fiber, magnesium, and calcium. In multivariate analysis, a 10 mmole increase in daily potassium intake was associated with a 40% reduction in the risk of stroke-associated mortality. This effect was independent of blood pressure and of other dietary variables, as well as of age, sex, blood cholesterol level, obesity, fasting blood glucose, and cigarette smoking. However, no data on discretionary sodium intake or supplementary potassium use were obtained. The authors conclude that a high intake of potassium from food sources may protect against stroke-associated death.

More recently, there has been increasing evidence on the role of fat consumption. Williams et al. [48] reported from a cross-sectional study that increased intake of monosaturated fat was related to lower levels of both systolic and diastolic blood pressure. Specifically, oleic acid and linoleic acid were responsible for these relationships.

The foregoing sections have illustrated that there are no clear answers about the role of specific nutrients in the etiology of hypertension. It is not likely that additional cross-sectional or even longitudinal studies will provide definitive answers.

When the associations found in the cross-sectional and prospective studies are consistent, persistent, and pertain to broad spectra of the population, it is appropriate to address the hypotheses so generated through interventional studies where the suspected nutrients are supplemented or restricted, to determine whether they can control or prevent hypertension. Such interventional studies or clinical trials must be large enough that if no differences are found, one can be sure that no effect really exists. If the clinical trials are too small, one can have little faith in the lack of a positive finding. It is encouraging that, increasingly, investigators and funding agencies are cognizant of the importance of designing studies with sufficient power to demonstrate differences between therapies.

WEIGHT CHANGE

In contrast to the evidence concerning nutrient components of food, the case for weight reduction in the control of hypertension is very strong.

Epidemiological evidence as well as clinical trials have confirmed that weight is an important factor in high blood pressure. Several prospective studies are worth noting. The Normative Aging Study, a longitudinal study of the Veterans Administration established in 1961, enrolled 2,280 men aged 21 to 81 years. Borcan [49] reports on 1,396 men who had a follow-up examination of at least 12 years after initial exam. The independent variable was percent change of body weight over that time interval. Those who had greater than a 10% weight loss had a reduction in systolic blood pressure of 6.5 mmHg, while those who had a greater than 10% gain had an increase in systolic blood pressure of 7.4 mmHg. Thus, there was a difference of about 14 mmHg in systolic blood pressure among the losers vs. the gainers. The decrease in diastolic blood pressure for those who lost weight was 6.9 and the increase for the gainers was 3.0, with a difference of about 10 mmHg between the losers and the gainers.

The Framingham offspring 8-year follow-up study reported by Helen Hubert [50] describes the life-style and behavioral correlates of change in coronary heart disease risk factors measured at 8-year follow-up in the young adult offspring of the Framingham heart study cohort. Of 397 men and 497 women aged 20 to 29 at entry into the study, the attribute most strongly and consistently related to both lipoprotein and blood pressure changes in both sexes was change in body mass. Weight gain and increase in alcohol consumption in men and beginning oral contraceptive use in women were associated with increases in blood pressure over the study period. A particularly relevant study by Henry Noppa [51] investigated the relationship between body weight and weight change in relation to incidence of ischemic heart disease and in relation to the change in risk factors for ischemic heart disease. In this study, 1,302 women were followed for six years. Seventy-five percent of the cohort were between 46 and 60 years of age at the initial examination. Noppa found a significant correlation between weight gain and the incidence of hypertension and of angina; these correlations persisted after adjustment for initial body weight. There was a significant correlation between change in body weight and change in arterial blood pressure, which persisted after adjustment for initial body weight. Thus, both obesity and weight change appear to be important factors.

In the Hypertension Detection and Follow-up Program (HDFP), over 10,000 participants with diastolic blood pressure of 90 mmHg were randomized into either a stepped-care group treated pharmacologically in specially set up HDFP clinics or a referred-care group of patients who were referred back to their usual sources of care [52,53]. In this study, the stepped-care regimen resulted in a lowering of systolic and diastolic blood pressure and a resultant decrease in morbidity and mortality. Of note, however, is that the decrease in both systolic and diastolic pressure was virtually linearly related to the amount of weight lost by the participants in both the stepped- and the referred-care group. Thus, weight reduction potentiated the effect of pharmacological therapy in the HDPF participants.

A variety of intervention studies have also shown that weight loss is important in controlling high blood pressure. The DISH [54] study found that participants in the weight-reduction treatment group were 3.5 times more likely to remain off medication for over a year, after controlling for other confounding variables, than were those in the control group. A study by Rissanen [55] of a group of 64 obese hypertensives in Helsinki who were enrolled in a 12-month program focused on weight reduction, salt restriction, or a combination of both. At 12 months, blood pressure was improved in 67% of the weight-reduction group, 61% of the weight- and salt-reduction combined group, and in only 12% of the salt-reduction group. The authors concluded that blood pressure control is strongly related to weight loss but not to reduced sodium excretion. These results have also been shown in the TAIM study, in which weight reduction was beneficial in lowering blood pressure and enhanced the blood-pressure-lowering effect of drugs, while sodium restriction was not found to be useful [56].

SUMMARY

Taking all the evidence together, what then is the state of our knowledge about the specific nutrients and their role in high blood pressure? The evidence for the role of sodium, both from cross-sectional and longitudinal studies is mixed. There appears to be some association but it is weak in intra-societal studies and most likely confounded by other variables in inter-societal studies. Nevertheless, several large clinical trials of intervention with sodium restriction, both for the control and prevention of hypertension have been conducted. The Dietary Intervention Study of Hypertension (DISH) [44,45] previously mentioned and the Hypertension Control Program [57] both have compared participants randomized to a sodium restriction group with those who had usual diet. In both these studies, the participants randomized to treatment had previously been treated pharmacologically for a period of over five years and were withdrawn from drug therapy before being placed on a dietary regimen. Thus, the findings from these studies have limited applicability to the large population of mild hypertensives with newly diagnosed hypertension. Both these studies found that a greater proportion of individuals assigned to sodium restriction could remain off drugs for a longer period of time than their comparison group. However, in the Dietary Intervention Study of Hypertension, we found that of the patients assigned to the sodium restriction group, approximately 60% were able to reduce their urinary sodium excretion to less than 100 mEq and of that group who were successful in reducing their sodium intake, 54% were able to remain drug free for at least 56 weeks with their blood pressure under control. But of those who were not able to reduce their sodium intake to that level, 56% also remained drug-free [58]. Multivariate analysis showed that no one factor was able to predict who would respond to the sodium-restriction intervention by not needing drugs. Thus, since both those who were successful in the intervention and those who were not successful in the intervention showed similar blood pressure effects from the sodium-restriction regimen compared with controls, these findings raised the possibility that factors other than sodium reduction affected blood pressure response for those in the sodium-restriction group. Furthermore, in DISH, sodium restriction for obese participants was not effective, while weight reduction was. In the Hypertension Control Program, the intervention group included sodium restriction, weight reduction, and alcohol reduction, and while sodium restriction seemed to have a benefit, it was not possible to separate out its effects from the effects of the other dietary modifications. Thus, these clinical trials have not fully answered the question of the effectiveness of sodium restriction.

While there are other studies still in progress that seek to determine whether sodium restriction can be used to control the blood pressure of mildly hypertensive patients, there are currently no data from clinical trials which indicate that sodium restriction is unequivocally a useful treatment modality. Thus, the case for sodium restriction appears to be weaker than it was once thought to be, and the evidence is not in for changing the entire diet of the United States population. However, it is likely that there are some individuals who are salt sensitive. In the DISH study, we were not able to identify a priori what characterized those individuals who would respond to the sodium-restriction regimen. More research is needed to identify individuals who are likely to benefit by sodium restriction.

With regard to calcium, again the evidence from both cross-sectional and prospective trials is conflicting and does not offer convincing proof that high-calcium diet or that calcium supplementation can control blood pressure. The intervention trials that have been done using calcium supplementation have generally used small numbers of individuals. The state of the art concerning calcium is that more prospective studies are needed, and if they provide more convincing evidence about dietary calcium, then larger clinical trials would be warranted.

With regard to dietary potassium, the evidence of its role in preventing or controlling hypertension is highly suggestive. Most of the research done with potassium has been confounded with sodium restriction, and at this point it would be useful to have elegantly designed, shorter-term studies of potassium supplementation.

The role of alcohol is quite clear. Alcohol intake has an adverse effect on blood pressure. The role of polyunsaturated fats, magnesium, and vitamins A and C are all in early stages of investigation. The point is that it will continue to be very difficult to separate out the roles of specific nutrients. Thus, a prudent diet with high quantities of fruit and vegetables is a reasonable approach.

In summary, nutrition is clearly related to blood pressure. There is little disagreement about that. However, the extent of the role of specific nutrients is not firmly established. Weight and body-mass index, however, are clearly epidemiologically related to hypertension, and weight loss for the overweight appears to be an effective way to lower blood pressure in a large proportion of mildly hypertensive individuals and likely to be an effective preventive modality for the general population.

REFERENCES

Morgan RW, Jain M, Miller AB, Choi NW, Matthews V, Munan L, Burch JD, Feather J, Howe GR, Kelly A (1978): A comparison of dietary methods in epidemiologic studies. Am J Epidemiol 107(6):488–498.

Jain M, Howe G.R, Johnson K.C., Miller A.B. (1980): Evaluation of a diet history questionnaire for epidemiologic studies. Am J Epidemiol 111(2):212–219.

Rohan, T.E., Potter J.D. (1984): Retrospective assessment of dietary intake. Am J Epidemiol 120(6):876–887.

Block G. (1982): A review of validations of dietary assessment methods. Am J Epidemiol 115(4):492–505.

Dawber T.R., Pearson G., Anderson P., et al. (1962): Dietary assessment in the epidemiologic study of coronary heart disease: The Framingham Study. II. Reliability of measurement. Am J Clin Nutr 11:226–234.

Reshef A., Epstein L.M. (1972): Reliability of a dietary questionnaire. Am J Clin Nutr 25:91–95.

Liu K., Stamler J., Dyer A., McKeever J., McKeever P. (1978): Statistical methods to assess and minimize the role of intra-individual variability in obscuring the relationship between dietary lipids and serum cholesterol. J Chron Dis 31:399–418.

Sempos C.T., Johnson N.E., Smith E.L., Gilligan C. (1985): Effects of intraindividual and interindividual variation in repeated dietary records. Am J Epidemiol 121(1):120–130.

Beaton G.H., Milner J., Corey P., McGuire V., Cousins M., Stewart E., de Ramos M., Hewitt D., Grambsch P.V., Kassim N., Little J.A. (1979): Sources of variance in 24-hour dietary recall data: Implications for nutrition study design and interpretation. Am J Clin Nutr 32:2546–2559.

Reed D., McGee D., Yano K., Hankin J. (1985): Diet, Blood pressure and multicollinearity. Hypertension 7(3):405–410.

McCarron D.A., Morris C.D. Evidence for a Protective Action of the Cation. In: Calcium and Hypertension. pp 167–186.

McCarron D.A., Stanton J., Henry H., Morris C. (1983): Assessment of nutritional correlates of blood pressure. Ann Intern Med 98(2):715–719.

McCarron D.A., Morris C.D., Henry H.J., Stanton J.L. (1984): Blood pressure and nutrient intake in the United States. Science 224:1392–1398.

Gruchow H.W., Sobocinski K.A., Barboriak J.J. (1985): Alcohol, nutrient intake and hypertension in US adults. JAMA 253(11):1567–1570.

McCarron D.A. (1985): Is calcium more important than sodium in the pathogenesis of essential hypertension? Hypertension 7(4):607–626.

MacGregor G.A. (1985): Sodium is more important than calcium in essential Hypertension. Hypertension 7(4):628–640.

Dahl L.K., Love R.A. (1954): Evidence for relationship between sodium (chloride) intake and human essential hypertension. AMA Arch Intern Med 94:525–530.

Joossens J.V., Geboers J. (1983): Salt and hypertension. Prev Med 12:53–59.

Intersalt Cooperative Research Group (1988): Intersalt: an international study of electrolyte excretion and blood pressure. Results for 24 hour urinary sodium and potassium excretion. Br Med J 297:319–328.

Smith WCS, Crombie I.K., Tavendale R.T., et al. (1988): Urinary electrolyte excretion, alcohol consumption, and blood pressure in the Scottish Heart Health Study. Br Med J 297:329–330.

Sempos C., Cooper R., Kovar M.G., Johnson C., Drizd T., Yetley E. (1986): Dietary calcium and blood pressure in National Health and Nutrition Examination Surveys I and II. Hypertension 8(11):1067–1074.

Schramm M.M., Cauley J.A., Sandler R.B., Slemenda C.W. (1986): Lack of an association between calcium intake and blood pressure in postmenopausal women. Am J Clin Nutr 44:505–511.

Kok F.J., Vandenbroucke J.P., van der Heide-Wessel C., van der Heide R.M. (1986): Dietary sodium, calcium and potassium, and blood pressure. Am J Epidemiol 123(6):1043–1048.

Kaplan N.M., Meese R.B. (1986): The calcium deficiency hypothesis: A critique. Ann Intern Med 105:947–955.

Keys A., Menotti A., Karvonen M.J., Aravanis C., Blackburn H., Buzina R., Djordjevic B.S., Donatas A.S., Fidanza F., Keys M.H., Kromhaut D., Nedeljkovic S., Punsar S.,

Seccareccia F., Toshima H. (1986): The diet and 15-year death rate in the Seven Countries Study. Am J Epidemiol 124(6):903–915.

Kromhaut D., Bosschieter E.B., de Lezenne Coulander C. (1985): Potassium, calcium, alcohol intake and blood pressure: the Zutphen Study. Am J Clin Nutr 41:1299–1304.

Joffres M.R., Reed D.M., Yano K. (1987): Relationship of magnesium intake and other dietary factors to blood pressure: the Honolulu Heart Study. Am J Clin Nutr 45:469–475.

Kannel W.B., Sorlie P. (1974): Hypertension in Framingham. In: O. Paul (ed): "Epidemiology and Control of Hypertension." New York: Grune and Stratton, pp 553–592.

D'Alonzo C.A., Pell S. Cardiovascular diseases among problem drinkers. J Occup Med 10:334–350.

Myrhed M. (1974): Blood Pressure. In "Alcohol Consumption in Relation to Factors Associated with Ischemic Heart Disease." Acta Med Scand (suppl) 567:40–46.

Mitchell, P.I., Morgan M.J., Boadle D.J., et al. (1980): Role of alcohol in the aetiology of hypertension. Med J Aust 2:198–200.

Bulpitt C.J., Shipley M.J., Semmence A.M. (1981): Blood Pressure and Alcohol Intake. Abstr. presented 9th Int. Scientific Meeting, Int. Epidemiol. Assoc., Edinburgh, August 22–28.

Geboers J., Bellens A., Kesteloot H. (1982): Alcohol, Gamma-glutamyl-transpeptidase and blood pressure. CVD Epidemiol Newsletter No. 31:40.

Arkwright P.D., Beilin L.J., Rouse I., et al. (1982): Effects of alcohol use and other aspects of lifestyle on blood pressure levels and prevalence of hypertension in a working population. Circulation 66:60–66.

Barboriak P.N., Anderson A.J., Hoffmann R.G., Barboriak J.J. (1982): Blood pressure and alcohol intake in heart patients. Clin Exp Res 6:234–238.

Fortmann S.P., Haskell W.L., Vranizan K., et al. (1983): The association of blood pressure and dietary alcohol: Differences by age, sex, and estrogen use. Am J Epidemiol 118:497–507.

Cooke K.M., Frost G.W., Thornell I.R., Stokes G.S. (1982): Alcohol consumption and blood pressure: Survey of the relationship at a health-screening clinic. Med J Aust 1:65–69.

Klatsky A.L., Friedman G.D., Siegelaub A.B., Gerard M.J. (1977): Alcohol consumption and blood pressure: Kaiser-Permanente Multiphasic Health Examination data. N Engl J Med 296:1194–1200.

Miller J.M., Miller J.M. (1986): Association of hypertension with chronic alcoholism. J Natl Med Assoc 78:391–393.

Criqui M.H., Wallace R.B., Mishkel M., Barret-Connor E., Heiss G. Alcohol consumption and blood pressure. The Lipid Research Clinics Prevalence Study. Hypertension 3:557–565.

Usehima H., Shimamoto T., Lida T., et al. (1984): Alcohol intake and hypertension among urban and rural Japanese population. J Chron Dis 37:585–592.

Weissfeld J.L., Johnson E.H., Brock B.M., Hawthorn V.M. (1988): Sex and age interaction in the association between alcohol and blood pressure. Am J Epidemiol 128(3):559–569.

Potter J.F., Beevers D.G. (1984): Pressor effect of alcohol in hypertension. Lancet 1:119–122.

Langford, H.G. (1987): Potassium and its role in the etiology and therapy of hypertension. Biblthca Cardiol 41:57–68.

Langford H.G., Blaufox M.D., Oberman A., Hawkins C.M., Curb J.D., Cutter G.R., Wassertheil-Smoller S., Pressel S., Babcock C., Abernathy J.D., Hotchkiss J., Tyler M. (1985): Dietary therapy slows the return of hypertension after stopping prolonged medication. JAMA 253:657–664.

Wassertheil-Smoller S., Langford H.G., Blaufox M.D., Oberman A., Hawkins M., Levine B., Cameron M., Babcock C., Pressel S., Caggiula A., Cutter G., Curb D., Wing R.

(1985): Effective dietary intervention in hypertensives: Sodium restriction and weight reduction. JAMA 85(4):423–430.

Khaw K.-T., Barrett-Connor E. (1987): Dietary potassium and stroke-associated mortality: A 12-year prospective population study. N Engl J Med 316(5):235–240.

Williams P.T., Fortmann S.P., Terry R.B., Garay S.C., Vranizan K.M., Ellsworth N., Wood P.D. (1987): Associations of dietary fat, regional adiposity and blood pressure in men. JAMA 257(23):3251–3256.

Borkan G.A., Sparrow D., Wisniewski C., Volkonas P.S. (1986): Body weight and coronary disease risk: Patterns of risk factor change associated with long-term weight change. The Normative Aging Study. Am J Epidemiol 124(3):410–419.

Hubert H.B., Eaker E.D., Garrison R.J., Castelli W.P. (1987): Lifestyle Correlates of Risk Factor Change in Young Adults: An Eight-Year Study of Coronary Heart Disease Risk Factors in the Framingham Offspring. Am J Epidemiol 125(5):812–831.

Noppa H. (1980): Body weight change in relation to incidence of ischemic heart disease and change in risk factors for ischemic heart disease. Am J Epidemiol 111:693–704.

HDFP Cooperative Group (1979): Five-Year Findings of the Hypertension Detection and Follow-Up Program I. Reduction in Mortality of Persons with High Blood Pressure Including Mild Hypertension. JAMA 343:2562–2571.

HDFP Cooperative Group (1982): The Effect of Treatent on Mortality in "Mild" Hypertension, Results of the Hypertension Detection and Follow-Up Program. N Engl J Med 307:976–980.

Balufox M.D., Langford H.G., Oberman A., Hawkins C.M., Curb J.D., Cutter G.R., Wassertheil-Smoller S., Pressel S., Babcock C., Abernathy J.D., Hotchkiss J., Tyler M. (1985): Dietary Intervention Study of Hypertension (DISH). Cardiov Rev Rep 6(9):1036–1052.

Rissanen A., Pietinen P., Siljamaki-Ojansuu U., Piirainen H., Reissel P. (1985): Treatment of hypertension in obese patients: Efficacy and feasibility of weight and salt reduction programs. Acta Med Scand 218:149–156.

Langford H.G., Davis B.R., Oberman A., Blaufox M.D., Smoller S.W., Hawkins C.M., Zimbaldi N., Rosett J.W. for the TAIM Study Group (1989): The TAIM Study: Diet-Drug Combinations in the Treatment of Mild Hypertension. Abstract of the 2nd International Conference on Preventive Cardiology and the 29th Annual Meeting of the AHA Council on Epidemiology, Washington, D.C., June 18–22.

Stamler R., Stamler J., Grimm R., Gosch F.C., Elmer P., Dyer A., R. Berman, J. Fishman, N. VanHeel, J. Civinelli, A. McDonald (1987): nutritional therapy for high blood pressure: Final report of a four-year randomized controlled trial—The Hypertension Control Program. JAMA 257(11):1484–1491.

Wassertheil-Smoller S., Balufox M.D., Langford H.G., Oberman A., Cutter G., Pressel S. (1986): Prediction of response to sodium intervention for blood pressure control. J Hyperten 4 (suppl):S343–S346.

Nutritional Factors in Hypertension
© *1990 Alan R. Liss, Inc., pages 35–50*

3 | Alcohol and Hypertension

Howard S. Friedman, M.D.

INTRODUCTION

Since 1915, when Lian reported alcoholism as a cause of hypertension in French servicemen, alcohol use has been related to elevations of systemic blood pressure. Although numerous epidemiologic studies have demonstrated relationships between alcohol consumption and an increased blood pressure, a causal association has eluded confirmation until recently. The reluctance to accept these population findings was related, in part, to the known vasodilator actions of alcohol and its metabolites. In fact, in healthy humans, ingestion of alcohol generally produces a decline in systemic arterial resistance with an increase of cardiac output, but without a consistent effect on arterial blood pressure. The finding of an increased blood pressure in alcoholics undergoing detoxification has suggested that alcohol withdrawal, with its profound sympathoadrenal effects, might be responsible for the epidemiologic observations relating alcohol use to elevations of blood pressure. However, recent studies have demonstrated that the ingestion of large amounts of alcohol for several weeks in healthy subjects will elevate arterial blood pressure. Other studies have shown that hypertensive alcoholics may become normotensive with abstinence—and may even lose their requirements for antihypertensive drugs—but will become hypertensive soon after resumption of alcohol use. Also, a study in experimental animals has shown

From the Section of Cardiology, the Department of Medicine, The Brooklyn Hospital and the SUNY Health Science Center, 121 DeKalb Avenue, Brooklyn, NY, 11201.

a similar blood pressure response when alcohol was added to the diet. These findings are not only of importance to the general population—with implications for the contribution of alcohol use to the prevalence of hypertension—but may be important in understanding the biomedical complications of alcohol abuse: stroke, myocardial infarction, and congestive heart failure, known consequences of hypertension, are indeed serious problems that ensue in the alcoholic. This chapter will review the epidemiologic, clinical, and laboratory investigations relating alcohol to blood pressure and the implications of those findings.

EPIDEMIOLOGIC STUDIES

Numerous studies have demonstrated in diverse populations that alcohol use elevates systemic blood pressure independent of the confounding influence of age, body weight, or cigarette smoking. Moreover, systemic hypertension has been found to be more prevalent with use, and especially with abuse, of alcohol. The findings of representative epidemiologic studies are summarized in Table 1. The relation of alcohol and blood pressure has generally been found to be linear, but curvilinear associations, especially in women [27,30,36,54], U-shaped curves [33], and even the absence of a consistent [16] pattern have been reported. As the table indicates, the findings are present in both men and women, albeit with stronger associations generally, but not always [17], found in men.

Although alcohol use has been related to both systolic and diastolic pressures, the influence of alcohol appears to be greater on the systolic value. However, by contrast to the independent effects of age and adiposity on blood pressure, the contribution of alcohol use seems to be relatively small, with multivariate regression coefficients of less than 0.10 generally found. Even so, the impact is such that alcohol use can be related to an increased prevalence of hypertension [5,8,11,28,42,44] and, moreover, in a longitudinal study, heavy drinking has been shown to increase the risk of developing hypertension [19].

A controversy, still unsettled, is whether a "threshold" exists at which alcohol consumption leads to an elevation of blood pressure. Some studies have even suggested a dip in blood pressure for light alcohol usage, producing U- or J-shaped relationships. In the Tecumseh Community Health Study, Harburg et al. [30] found lower blood pressures in light drinkers than in abstainers with the trough in the curve occurring at 1½ drinks per week for men and at 4 drinks per week for women; an increased blood pressure was evident in men with 1 to 2 drinks per day, but more than 5 drinks per day were required in women. Similar findings were obtained in the Framingham Study: the trough for adjusted systolic blood pressure occurred at about 1

TABLE 1. Epidemiologic Studies Relating Alcohol Use to Systemic Blood Pressure

Authors	Year	Country	Males	Females	Systolic pressure	Diastolic	Linear	Threshold effect	Independent variable
Arkwright et al.	1982	Australia	Yes	NS	Yes	No	Yes	No	Yes
Cairns et al.	1984	Germany	Yes	Yes	Yes	Yes	Yes	No	Yes
Coates et al.	1984	Canada	No	No	No	No	No	No	No
Cooke et al.	1982	Australia	Yes	Yes	Yes	Yes	Yes	No	Yes
Fortmann et al.	1983	USA	Yes	Yes*	Yes	Yes	Yes	No	Yes
Gyntelberg and Meyer	1974	Denmark	Yes	NS	Yes	Yes	Yes	No	Yes
Harburg et al.	1980	USA	Yes	Yes	Yes	Yes	No+	Yes	Yes
Gordon and Kannel	1983	USA	Yes	Yes	Yes	Yes	No†	Yes	Yes
Jackson et al.	1985	New Zealand	Yes	Yes	Yes	Yes	No§	No	Yes
Klatsky et al.	1986	USA	Yes	Yes	Yes	Yes	Yes+	No ψ	Yes
Kondo and Ebihara	1984	Japan	Yes	No	Yes	Yes	Yes	Yes	Yes
Kromhout et al.	1985	Netherlands	Yes	NS	Yes	Yes	Yes	No	Yes
MacMahon et al.	1984	Australia	Yes	Yes ¶	Yes	Yes	Yes	No	Yes
Milon et al.	1982	France	Yes	No	Yes	Yes	Yes	No	Yes
Paulin et al.	1985	New Zealand	Yes	No	Yes	Yes	Yes	No	Yes
Savdie et al.	1984	Australia	Yes	Yes	Yes	Yes	Yes	No	Yes
Ueshima et al.	1984	Japan	Yes	No	Yes	Yes	Yes	No	Yes
Wallace et al.	1982	USA	NS	Yes	Yes	Yes	No+	No	Yes

NS, not studied; *, Older women (50–75 years); +, curvilinear for women; †, curvilinear for men and women; §, U-shaped relation; ψ, at 1 to 2 drinks per day change evident; ¶, borderline statistical significance.

drink per day in men and 4 to 5 drinks per day in women, with greater than 5 drinks per day required for an increased adjusted systolic blood pressure. In the Lipid Research Clinical Prevalence Study, [54] the lowest blood pressure in women was observed at less than 2 drinks per week and an increased value was not evident at less than 3 drinks per day. Kondo and Ebihara [37] found in a rural community in Japan no dip in blood pressure with light drinking, but 1 to 2 drinks per day were required to elevate blood pressure in men. In the Kaiser-Permanente Study, Klatsky et al. [35] found that a fall in blood pressure was evident in women who drank 2 or fewer drinks per day; in 1986, Klatsky et al. [36] reported, however, that as few as 1 to 2 drinks per day elevates blood pressure in both men and women.

The discrepancy between these studies and those that failed to identify a dip or a threshold might be related to differences in group categorization and to the impact of confounding factors. For instance, in the study by Cooke et al. [17] the range for light usage was taken as 1 to 10 drinks per week, the upper limit exceeding the amount reported to be associated with a blood pressure lowering effect. In the Tecumseh Community Health Study [30] adjustment for age and body weight was shown to lessen the apparent dip in blood pressure observed in women who were light drinkers. Studies by Cooke et al. [17], MacMahon et al. [42], and Milon et al. [44] have confirmed that correction for age and adiposity makes the dip disappear. Also, it is unlikely that 1 to 2 drinks per week would have a long-term physiological effect on blood pressure, supporting the perception that light drinkers may have other characteristics that influence blood pressure.

Not only has there been controversy regarding the presence of a threshold for the hypertensive effects of alcohol, but there are also data that suggest a plateau. Several studies [17,36,52] have shown that the blood pressure elevating effects of alcohol levels off at approximately 9 drinks per day. Whether this is merely a statistical artifact, as suggested by Klatsky et al. [36], is not clear. Certainly, the myriad of biomedical and psychosocial factors present in the alcoholic are likely to confound a simple linear relation.

Other factors that might influence the impact of alcohol consumption on blood pressure include type of beverage used, race, and age. As shown in Table 1, the relation is not limited to any national group. The association of alcohol use and blood pressure is observed in countries where the preferred beverage may be beer, wine, saki, or whisky. Although Klatsky et al. [36] found a continuous relation of alcohol use and blood pressure in black men, this relation was weaker than that found in Caucasians. At least two studies [37,53] have demonstrated blood pressure elevating effects of alcohol in Japanese men. Also, there is evidence that older persons—those more than fifty years old—may have an increased sensitivity to the blood pressure elevating effects of alcohol [8,21,36,44]. Fortmann et al. [21] observed that this finding in older women was less evident in those receiving supplemental estrogens, suggesting a modulating influence of hormones on this effect.

Although epidemiological surveys have demonstrated a link between alcohol use and elevation of blood pressure, there are concerns regarding the significance of this observation. First, the findings have not been consistent in all studies. This may be related in part to the impact of confounding factors. Obesity and cigarette smoking are two such influences. Obesity correlates positively with both alcohol use and blood pressure, whereas cigarette smoking correlates positively with alcohol use but negatively with blood pressure. Consequently, in multivariate analyses that include these variables, the relation of alcohol use to blood pressure is affected. Also, the interdependence of such factors may be so strong that by mathematically controlling the influence, the relationship might be obscured. For instance, in women alcohol abuse may be strongly associated with the abuse of other substances. By controlling for this effect, the size of the subgroup of alcoholic women who are not addicts becomes too small in most studies to demonstrate statistically significant findings. Moreover, because of the relatively small contribution of alcohol to elevation of blood pressure in general, in populations, such as Japan, where alcohol use is not prevalent, and if used, generally in small amounts, the impact of alcohol on blood pressure might not be evident. This might account for the absence of a relation of alcohol use and blood pressure in women that has been reported in some studies.

Another limitation of these population studies is that the estimates of alcohol use have generally been based on questionnaire responses. Because of the tendency to underestimate alcohol use, the amount imbibed to produce the blood pressure changes reported may be greater than these studies would suggest. However, the repeated findings of linear or curvilinear relationships and the absence of such an association in past drinkers of alcohol [5] would support a causal link. Moreover, studies of alcoholics in which use of alcohol has been related to biochemical markers, such as serum levels of gamma glutamyltransferase [10], have also shown a linear relation of alcohol use to the level of systemic blood pressure. Thus, despite the limitations inherent in epidemiological studies and the problem of confounding influences, the body of evidence from population studies supports a positive relation of alcohol use to systemic blood pressure and an increased prevalence of systemic hypertension in alcohol abusers.

HYPERTENSION OF ALCOHOL DETOXIFICATION

Alcohol withdrawal is characterized by an intense psychomotor and sympathoadrenal reaction. Not surprisingly, hypertension is frequently observed

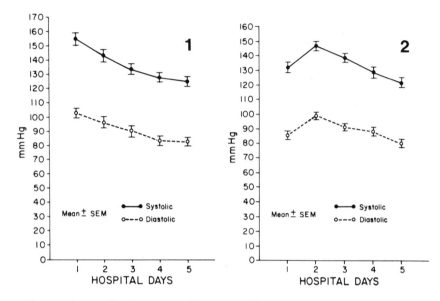

Fig. 1. Average blood pressures in 48 patients with transitory hypertension, having highest blood pressures on admission with a gradual decline over 5 days. (Reprinted with permission from Clark et al., *Alcoholism: Clinical and Experimental Research* 9:127, 1985).

Fig. 2. Average blood pressures in 12 patients with transitory hypertension having highest blood pressures on 2nd or 3rd hospital day. (Reprinted with permission from Clark et al., *Alcoholism: Clinical Experimental Research* 9:127, 1985).

in this setting. Beevers et al. [10] found that 50% of alcoholics undergoing detoxification had a systolic pressure greater than 140 mmHg or a diastolic pressure greater than 90 mmHg or both; Mehta and Sereny [43a] observed that 40% of such patients had a systolic pressure greater than 160 mmHg or a diastolic pressure greater than 95 mmHg or both; and Clark and Friedman [14] found, in a study of alcoholics undergoing detoxification but with those having delirium tremens excluded, that 33% had the blood pressure elevations reported by Mehta and Sereny [43a]. Although the peak blood pressures in such patients were generally observed on the day of admission for detoxification, in 20% of those with hypertension, the peak occurred on the second or third day. In most of the hypertensives blood pressure gradually declined to normotensive values. These responses are displayed in Figures 1 and 2. However, even after all features of withdrawal had abated, 9% of the alcoholics still had systemic hypertension [14,51], a value that probably reflects the prevalence of nonalcoholic-associated hypertension in this population. Also, alcoholics whose blood pressure returned to normal values still showed

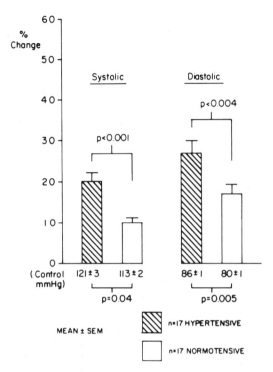

Fig. 3. Percent changes of blood pressure with cold pressor test. Increment in hypertensives is greater than in normotensives. (Reprinted with permission from Clark et al., *Alcoholism: Clinical Experimental Research* 9:129, 1985).

an exaggerated blood pressure response to a cold pressor test administered on the fourth or fifth hospital day (see Fig. 3).

The blood pressure response during alcohol detoxification has been related to withdrawal symptoms and to estimated recent use of alcohol or biochemical markers of such use. Beevers et al. [10] found that age/sex adjusted blood pressures had a linear relation to severity of withdrawal symptoms. These investigators also found a correlation of blood pressure with estimated daily intake of alcohol during the three months preceding detoxification; moreover, blood pressure correlated with markers of recent alcohol use, such as gamma glutamyltransferase and mean corpuscular volume after exclusion of cirrhotics. In an earlier study Saunders et al. [14] found that alcoholics with fatty liver and well-compensated cirrhosis had higher blood pressures than those with no histologic evidence of liver damage. By contrast, cirrhotics with ascites, jaundice, or varices had the lowest blood pressures, both during and after detoxification. The confounding influence of advanced liver disease on blood pressure—with the presence of arteriovenous shunts and increased blood levels of vasodilators, producing a reduced systemic resistance—has been known for some time [20].

Peak blood pressure and blood pressure response during withdrawal have been related to age of the alcoholic. Alcoholics with hypertension were observed to be older than those not showing this finding [9,14]. Moreover, persistence of hypertension after withdrawal was most commonly found in older alcoholics (greater than 50 years of age), whereas the lowest blood pressure and the pattern of a progressive decline in blood pressures, as illustrated in Figure 1, were found in the youngest alcoholics [9].

Alcohol detoxification is associated with elevation of various hormones. Plasma renin activity, cortisol, and aldosterone have all been correlated with the severity of withdrawal [7]. However, only plasma cortisol has been related, and then weakly, to blood pressure after alcohol withdrawal [7]. Bannan et al. [7] observed also that urine volume and 24 hour sodium excretion were diminished and that the 24-hour urine value varied inversely with diastolic pressure.

Increased blood and urinary catecholamines have been found on acute ingestion [32], with chronic use [45] and after withdrawal of alcohol [45]. Elevations of epinephrine and its metabolites are especially increased during alcohol detoxification [14], Clark and Friedman [14] found high average blood levels of epinephrine in both hypertensive and normotensive alcoholics undergoing detoxification; however, elevated blood epinephrine levels were more frequently observed in the hypertensives, with 86% having this finding, whereas only 44% of the normotensives. Moreover, hypertensives, at a time when blood pressure was normal and withdrawal symptoms had abated, demonstrated an exaggerated and atypical response to a cold pressor test (see Fig. 4). Not only did blood levels of norepinephrine increase after a cold pressor test, as observed in nonalcoholics [6,40], but plasma epinephrine also increased after this stress—a finding not observed in nonalcoholics. Thus, hypertension during alcohol detoxification appears to be associated with enhanced adrenal cortical and medullary function. However, whether the increased adrenal activity is sufficient to explain hypertension during alcohol withdrawal is not entirely clear.

Other studies during alcohol detoxification include measurements of plasma electrolytes, including magnesium [14] and atrial natriuretic factor [15]; however, differences in hypertensives have not been found. Although increased plasma levels of certain prostaglandin metabolites have also been observed in alcoholic hypertensives, the relation of these substances to blood pressure is not clear [15]. Changes in vascular and baroreceptor responsiveness—important determinants of blood pressure—have not been reported in hypertensive alcoholics. By contrast, a comprehensive study of such re-

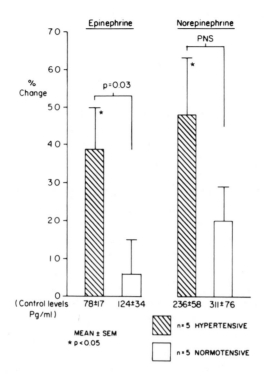

Fig. 4. Percent changes of catecholamines with cold pressor test. Increment of both plasma epinephrine and norepinephrine is significant only in hypertensives; also, percentage of increment of epinephrine is greater in hypertensives than in normotensives. (Reprinted with permission from Clark et al., *Alcoholism: Clinical Experimental Research* 9:129, 1985).

sponses, in which drinkers (1 or 2 drinks per day) with higher blood pressures were compared to nondrinkers, failed to disclose any differences [6].

CLINICAL STUDIES

Since 1984, clinical reports have appeared that have provided a conclusive link between alcohol use and elevation of systemic blood pressure. Potter and Beavers [47] studied the effects of continued drinking, withdrawal, and then resumption of alcohol in hypertensives who used on the average 60, but less than 80, grams per day. At the time of the investigation none had been receiving antihypertensive treatment for at least 2 weeks. Those given their estimated usual amount to drink showed no fall in blood pressure until alcohol was stopped, with a significant fall in systolic and diastolic blood pressure evident within 72 hours thereafter. Drinking a comparable amount of alcohol after 3 days of abstinence resulted, within 48 hours, in a significant elevation of blood pressure. These changes were evident in most, but not all, of the participants. Also, blood pressure effects were found to be accompanied by changes in plasma cortisol concentration but were not related to plasma renin activity, 24-hour urine volume, or 24-hour urinary sodium, potassium, or metanephrine.

A similar blood pressure response has been reported in normotensive users of alcohol (averaging approximately 3 drinks per day) who merely curtailed or resumed their normal use [48]. Male volunteers, averaging 35 years of age, were assigned either to a group that maintained a normal drinking pattern for 6 weeks followed by 6 weeks in which only a low alcohol content beer (0.9%, V/V) was permitted or to a group in which the same protocol was used but alcohol was first curtailed. By the second week of follow-up, a significant change in blood pressure was evident. Changes of systolic and diastolic pressure were found to correlate with both estimated use of alcohol and objective markers of alcohol consumption. However, on multivariate regression analysis, with weight change considered, only the relation of alcohol use with supine systolic blood pressure remained significant. Moreover, one-third of the participants did not show a fall in blood pressure on the low alcohol regimen. Despite the modest changes in blood pressure associated with alcohol use (1.1 mmHg of systolic pressure per drink/day), this study [48] demonstrated a direct effect of alcohol on blood pressure in a normotensive, nonalcoholic population that merely curtailed their use of alcohol.

Following the same protocol, Puddey et al. [49] examined the effects of alcohol intake on blood pressure in hypertensive, moderate to heavy drinkers (averaging 4 to 5 drinks per day). An estimated 85% reduction of alcohol use during the curtailment period produced significant decreases of systolic and diastolic pressures. These changes in blood pressure correlated with biochemical markers of alcohol use, and the findings were still evident after adjustment for weight changes. As this group observed in normotensive subjects [48], the independent effects of alcohol were modest, with less than 1 mmHg of blood pressure related to each drink per day.

Predilection for hypertension and recentness of exposure to alcohol may influence the effects of alcohol intake on blood pressure. Malhotra et al. [43] compared the effects of 5 days of 1 gm/kg of alcohol per day (approximately 5 to 6 drinks per day) to abstinence in volunteers: Normotensive light drinkers who had not used alcohol for the 2 weeks preceding the study showed no differences in blood pressure; hypertensive, light drinkers who had not taken alcohol or antihypertensive treatment for the 2 weeks preceding the study showed only higher standing blood pressures during the drinking period; whereas hypertensive, moderate drinkers who continued to drink their usual amount but had not taken antihypertensive treatment for the 2 weeks preceding the study showed higher standing and supine blood pressures during the drinking period. Thus hypertensives who use alcohol regularly might derive an especially beneficial effect from abstinence or even from curtailment of alcohol consumption.

EXPERIMENTAL STUDIES

Recently, Chan and Sutter [12] have reported that male Wistar rats given alcohol, as 20% (V/V) of drinking water, developed an increased blood pressure after 4 weeks of treatment. The increment of blood pressure was enhanced by chronic stress produced by 30 min per day of exposure to heat radiation [13]. Measurements obtained at 12 weeks showed that alcohol-treated animals had an increased plasma volume and a reduced 24-hour urine volume. Although plasma electrolytes were not different—except for perhaps a trend toward a lower plasma potassium concentration in the experimental group, alcohol-treated rats had a reduced urinary sodium concentration and an increase in both urinary calcium and magnesium concentrations. However, vascular responsiveness to catecholamines was not enhanced in aortic and portal vein strips obtained from these rats and, in fact, portal veins showed a reduced contractile response to norepinephrine in a bathing medium with a low calcium concentration. By contrast, alcohol treatment increased plasma norepinephrine levels. Moreover, the enhanced blood pressure response produced by chronic heat stress was associated with further elevation of plasma norepinephrine concentration but with no additional expansion in plasma volume.

Altura's group [1,2,4] has demonstrated, however, that changes in vascular responsiveness might indeed occur in rats after chronic ethanol treatment: Male Wistar rats given a liquid diet containing 6.8% (V/V) alcohol (control group received an equicaloric volume of a sucrose solution) for up to 24 months showed tolerance to the inhibitory effects of pharmacological concentrations of ethanol on spontaneous and evoked contractile responses of aortic and portal vein strips. Moreover, in a review Altura and Altura [4] have reported that alcohol-treated rats showed at 12 and 24 weeks enhanced evoked vascular contractions and that blood vessels obtained from these rats demonstrated dose-response curves consistent with the development of "supersensitivity." These changes in blood vessel reactivity were accompanied by an increased calcium and a decreased magnesium vascular content. Because these divalent cations are known modulators of contraction, such findings could explain the changes in vascular reactivity produced by chronic alcohol ingestion.

Thus, systemic hypertension has been produced in rats following chronic alcohol administration. Increased sympathetic activity—reflected by elevated plasma norepinephrine, sodium and water retention, and an enhanced excretion of calcium and magnesium—accompanies the elevation of blood pressure. Chronic stress, which can by itself lead to an increased blood pressure in rats, enhances the hypertensive and noradrenergic effects of alcohol. Other studies in rats given alcohol for up to 24 months have demonstrated also changes in blood vessel responsiveness and vascular divalent cation content. Further investigation is required, however, to determine whether these experimental models are indeed relevant to alcohol-associated hypertension in humans.

CLINICAL IMPLICATIONS

Hypertension is a risk factor for the occurrence of stroke, coronary heart disease, and congestive heart failure, disorders found with increased frequency in alcoholics. In a prospective, longitudinal study [18] and in a retrospective case-control investigation [26] the risk of stroke in moderate to heavy drinkers was 3 to 4 times that found in nondrinkers. The relative risk of stroke was not only related to estimates of alcohol use before the event but also to biochemical markers of such use [26]. Donahue et al. [18] observed, however, that the increased risk was only evident for hemorrhagic stroke. Although both of these studies reported that the risk was apparent even with the data adjusted for hypertension, Kozararevic et al. [38] found that the association of stroke and alcohol consumption lost its statistical significance when systolic pressure was included in a multivariate regression analysis. The increased risk of stroke may also be related to the effects of alcohol on cerebral blood flow [3,24] and coagulation [31], and to alcoholism-associated cardiovascular complications, with their attendant thromboembolic events [22].

Although alcohol use is generally viewed as a "protective influence" on development of coronary heart disease [34], a less widely recognized association is the increased risk of this disorder in problem drinkers [19,55]. Moreover, Dyer et al. [19] found that when blood pressure was considered in a multivariate analysis, the increased risk of coronary events associated with alcohol abuse was no longer evident. Thus alcohol abuse is associated with an increased incidence of coronary heart disease and this appears to be due, at least in part, to the development of hypertension.

Dilated cardiomyopathy is also a complication of alcohol abuse [22]. Despite numerous attempts, the features of this disorder have never been replicated in experimental animals [23]. Recently, Friedman et al. [25] observed that alcoholics who manifested hypertension during detoxification had worse systolic time indicies than alcoholics who did not have this finding

TABLE 2. Systolic Time Intervals in Normal Subjects and Hypertensive and Normotensive Alcoholics

	Normal (n = 10)	Hypertensive (n = 26)	Normotensive (n = 40)
PEP (ms)	86 ± 3	101 ± 2*	95 ± 2*
LVET (ms)	299 ± 5	257 ± 1*	273 ± 4*†
LVETI (ms)	418 ± 3	388 ± 4*	397 ± 3*
PEP/LVET	0.290 ± 0.01	0.398 ± 0.01*	0.350 ± 0.01*†

*p < 0.02 vs. normal subjects.
†p < 0.02 vs. hypertensive patients. Values are mean ± standard error of the mean.
LVET = left ventricular ejection time; LVETI = LVET index; PEP = preejection period. (Reprinted with permission from Friedman et al., *American Journal of Cardiology* 57:229, 1986.)

TABLE 3. Comparison of Matched Normotensive and Transitory Hypertensive Alcoholics

	Normotensive (n = 7)	Hypertensive (n = 7)
Age (yr)	34 ± 1	35 ± 2
Body surface area (m²)	1.9 ± 0.07	1.9 ± 0.07
Heart rate (beats/min)	73 ± 4	73 ± 5
Blood pressure (mmHg)	117 ± 3/77 ± 3	117 ± 3/78 ± 1
PEP/LVET	0.331 ± 0.014	0.415 ± 0.033*

*p < 0.05.
Values are mean ± standard error of the mean.
PEP/LVET = ratio of preejection period to left ventricular ejection time. (Reprinted with permission from Friedman et al., *Amercian Journal of Cardiology* 57:229, 1986.)

(Table 2). Moreover, this was evident even when blood pressure and heart rate had returned to normal values (Table 3). Hypertensive alcoholics also demonstrated features of left ventricular "hyperfunction," which has been suggested as a prodromal finding in hypertensives who develop congestive heart failure. Also, Chan and Sutter [13] have observed that rats developing hypertension after alcohol administration have a high incidence of circulatory congestion and death when exposed to an additional stress. Thus clinical and experimental evidence suggest that alcohol-associated hypertension might at least contribute to the development of congestive heart failure in alcoholics.

RECOMMENDATIONS

Alcohol consumption clearly influences blood pressure. Alcohol-associated hypertension may also contribute to the cardiovascular complications observed in alcoholics. Determining alcohol use is especially important in hypertensives. Because of the general tendency to underestimate alcohol intake, particular care should be taken in obtaining an accurate history of alcohol use. When alcohol abuse is suspected but denied, biochemical markers of alcohol abuse should be assessed. Because even 1 to 2 drinks per day may elevate blood pressure, especially in those with hypertension, hypertensives should be advised to use alcohol infrequently and then only in small amounts. Not only may alcoholism be the cause of hypertension, but the alcoholic is not likely to comply with recommendations for treatment. Alcohol-associated hypertension should therefore be regarded as a form of secondary hypertension that can be diagnosed without sophisticated testing and treated without surgery or drugs.

REFERENCES

1. Altura BT, Pohorecky LA, Altura BM (1980): Demonstration of tolerance to ethanol in non-nervous tissue: effects on vascular smooth muscle. Alcoholism: Clin Exp Res 4: 62–69.
2. Altura BM, Altura BT (1982): Microvascular and vascular smooth muscle actions of ethanol, acetaldehyde, and acetate. Fed Proc 41:2447–2451.
3. Altura BM, Altura BT, Gebrewald A (1983): Alcohol-induced spasms of cerebral blood vessels: relation to cerebrovascular accidents and sudden death. Science 220:331–333.
4. Altura BM, Altura BT (1987): Peripheral and cerebrovascular actions of ethanol, acetaldehyde, and acetate: relationship to divalent cations. Alcoholism: Clin Exp Res 11:99–111.
5. Arkwright PD, Beilin LJ, Rouse I, Armstrong BK, Vandongen R (1982): Effects of alcohol use and other aspects of lifestyle on blood pressure levels and prevalence of hypertension in a working population. Circulation 66:60–66.
6. Arkwright PD, Beilin LJ, Vandongen R, Rouse IA, Lalor C (1982): The pressor effect of moderate alcohol consumption in man: A search for mechanisms. Circulation 66:515–519.
7. Bannan LT, Potter JF, Beevers DG, Saunders JB, Walters JRF, Ingram MC (1984): Effect of alcohol withdrawal on blood pressure, plasma renin activity, aldosterone, cortisol and dopamine B-hydroxylase. Clin Sci 66:659–662.
8. Barboriak PN, Anderson AJ, Hoffmann RG, Barboriak JJ (1982): Blood pressure and alcohol intake in heart patients. Alcoholism: Clin Exp Res 6:234–238.
9. Beckman H, Frank RR, Robertson RS, Brady KA, Coin EJ (1981): Evaluation of blood pressure during early alcohol withdrawal. Ann Emerg Med 10:32–35.
10. Beevers DB, Bannan LT, Saunders JB, Paton A, Walters JRF (1982): Alcohol and hypertension. Contr Nephrol 30:92–97.
11. Cairns V, Ulrich K, Kleinbaum D, Doering A, Stieber J (1984): Alcohol consumption as a risk factor for high blood pressure. Hypertension 6:124–131.
12. Chan TCK, Sutter MC (1983): Ethanol consumption and blood pressure. Life Sci 33: 1965–1973.
13. Chan TCK, Wall RA, Sutter MC (1985): Chronic ethanol consumption, stress and hypertension. Hypertension 7:519–524.
14. Clark LT, Friedman HS (1985): Hypertension associated with alcohol withdrawal: assessment of mechanisms and complications. Alcoholism: Clin Exp Res 9:125–130.
15. Clark LT, Hoover EL, Crandall DL, Cervoni P, Haynes S, El Sherif N (1987): Atrial natriuretic peptide and postaglandin responses to alcohol induced hypertension. Clin Res (abstract) 35:440A.

16. Coates RA, Corey PN, Ashley MJ, Steele CA (1985): Alcohol consumption and blood pressure: analysis of data from the Canada health survey. Prev Med 14:1–14.

17. Cooke KM, Frost GW, Thornell IR, Stokes GS (1982): Alcohol consumption and blood pressure. Med J Aust 1:65–69.

18. Donahue RP, Abbott RD, Reed DM, Yano K (1986): Alcohol and hemorrhagic stroke. JAMA 255:2311–2314.

19. Dyer AR, Stamler J, Oglesby P, Berkson DM, Shekelle RB, Lepper MH, McKean H, Lindberg HA, Garside D, Tokich T (1981): Alcohol, cardiovascular risk factors and mortality: the Chicago experience. Circulation (suppl III) 64:20–27.

20. Fernando HA, Friedman HS (1976): Demonstration of the hyperdynamic heart of cirrhosis by echocardiography. Clin Res (abstract) 24:614A.

21. Fortmann SP, Haskell WL, Vranizan K, Brown BW, Farquhar JW (1983): The association of blood pressure and dietary alcohol: differences by age, sex and estrogen use. Am J Epidemiol 118:497–507.

22. Friedman HS, Geller SA, Lieber CS (1982): The effect of alcohol on the heart, skeletal muscle and smooth muscle. In Lieber CS (ed) Major Problems in Internal Medicine: Aspects of Alcoholism. Philadelphia PA, WB Saunders Chapter 11: pp 436–479.

23. Friedman HS, Lieber CS (1983): Alcohol and the heart. In Feldman E.B. (ed) Nutrition and Heart Disease. New York, N.Y. Churchill Livingston Chapter 8 pp 149–150.

24. Friedman HS, Lowery R, Archer M, Shaughnessy E, Scorza J (1984): The effects of ethanol on brain blood flow in awake dogs. J Cardiovasc Pharmacol, 6:344–348.

25. Friedman HS, Vasavada BC, Malec AM, Hassan KH, Shah A, Siddiqui S (1986): Cardiac function in alcohol-associated systemic hypertension. Am J Cardiol 57:227–231.

26. Gill JS, Zezulka AV, Shipley MJ, Gill SK, Beevers DG (1986): Stroke and alcohol consumption. N Engl J Med 315:1041–1046.

27. Gordon T, Kannel WB (1983): Drinking and its relation to smoking, blood pressure, blood lipids, and uric acid. Arch Intern Med 143:1366–1374.

28. Gruchow HW, Sobocinski KA, Barboriak JJ (1985): Alcohol, nutrient intake, and hypertension in US adults. JAMA 253:1567–1570.

29. Gyntelberg F, Meyer J (1974): Relationship between blood pressure and physical fitness, smoking and alcohol consumption in Copenhagen males aged 40–59. Acta Med Scand 195:375–380.

30. Harburg E, Ozgoren F, Hawthorne VM, Schork MA (1980): Community norms of alcohol usage and blood pressure: Tecumseh, Michigan. Am J Public Health 70:813–820.

31. Haut MJ, Cowan DH (1974): The effect of ethanol on hemostatic properties of human blood platelets. Am J Med 56:22–33.

32. Ireland MA, Vandongen R, Davidson L, Beilin LJ, Rouse IL (1984): Acute effects of moderate alcohol consumption on blood pressure and plasma catecholamines. Clin Sci 66:643–648.

33. Jackson R, Stewart A, Beaglehole R, Scragg R (1985): Alcohol consumption and blood pressure. Am J Epidemiol 122:1037–1044.

34. Kagan A, Yanko K, Rhoads GG, McGee DL (1981): Alcohol and cardiovascular disease: the Hawaiian experience. Circulation 64: (suppl III) 27–31.

35. Klatsky AL, Friedman GD; Siegelaub AB, Gerard MJ (1977): Alcohol consumption and blood pressure. N Engl J Med 296:1194–1200.

36. Klatsky AL, Friedman GD, Armstrong MA (1986): The relationships between alcoholic beverage use and other traits to blood pressure: a new Kaiser Permanente study. Circulation 73:628–636.

37. Kondo K, Ebihara A (1984): Alcohol consumption and blood pressure in a rural commu-

nity of Japan. In Walter Lovenberg (ed) Nutritional prevention of cardiovascular disease. Orlando, Florida Academic Press, Inc. pp 217–220.

38. Kozararevic D, Vojvodic N, Dawber T, McGee DM, Racic Z, Gordon T (1980): Frequency of alcohol consumption and morbidity and mortality. Lancet i 613–616.
39. Kromhout D, Bosschieter EB, Coulander CL (1985): Potassium, calcium, alcohol intake and blood pressure: the Zutphen study. Am J Clin Nutr 41:1299–1304.
40. Lennart A, Lennart H (1981): Circulatory effects of stress in essential hypertension. Acta Med Scand 646:69–72.
41. Lian C (1915): L'alcoholisme cause d'hypertension arterielle. Bull Acad Med (Paris) 74:525–528.
42. MacMahon S, Blacket RB, Macdonald GJ, Hall W (1984): Obesity, alcohol consumption and blood pressure in Australian men and women. The National Heart Foundation of Australia risk factor prevalence study. J Hypertension 2:85–91.
43. Malhotra H, Mathur D, Mehta SR, Khandelwal PD (1985): Pressor effects of alcohol in normotensive and hypertensive subjects. Lancet ii 584–586.
43a. Mehta B, Sereny G (1979): Cardiovascular manifestations during alcohol withdrawal. Mt Sinai J Med NY 46:484–486.
44. Milon H, Froment A, Gaspard P, Guidollet J, Ripoll JP (1982): Alcohol consumption and blood pressure in a French epidemiological study. Eur Heart J 3:59–64.
45. Orgata M, Mendelson JH, Mello NK, Majchrowicz E (1971): Adrenal function and alcoholism. Psychosomatic Med 33:159–178.
46. Paulin JM, Simpson FO, Waal-Manning HJ (1985): Alcohol consumption and blood pressure in a New Zealand community study. New Zeland Med J 98:425–429.
47. Potter JE, Beevers DG (1984): Pressor effect of alcohol in hypertension. Lancet i 119–122.
48. Puddey IB, Beilin LJ, Vandongen R, Rouse IL, Rogers P (1985): Evidence for a direct effect of alcohol consumption on blood pressure in normotensive men. Hypertension 7:707–713.
49. Puddey IB, Beilin LJ, Vandongen R (1987): Regular alcohol use raises blood pressure in treated hypertensive subjects. Lancet i 647–662.
50. Salonen JT, Tuomilehto J, Tanskanen A (1983): Relation of blood pressure to reported intake of salt, saturated fats, and alcohol in healthy middle-aged population. J Epidemiol Community Health. 37:32–37.
51. Saunders JB, Beevers DG, Paton A (1979): Factors influencing blood pressure in chronic alcohlics. Clin Sci 57:295s–298s.
52. Savdie E, Grosslight GM, Adena MA (1984): Relation of alcohol and cigarette consumption to blood pressure and serum creatinine levels. J Chron Dis 37:617–623.
53. Ueshima H, Shimamoto T, Iida M, Konishi M, Tanigaki M, Doi M, Tsujioka K, Nagano E, Tsuda C, Ozawa H, Kojima S, Komachi Y (1984): Alcohol intake and hypertension among urban and rural Japanese populations. J Chron Dis 37:585–592.
54. Wallace RB, Connor EB, Criqui M, Wahal P, Hoover J, Hunninghake D, Heiss G (1982): Alteration in blood pressures associated with combined alcohol and oral contraceptive use—the lipid research clinics prevalence study. J Chron Dis 35:251–257.
55. Wilhelmsen L, Wedel H, Tibblin G (1973): Multivariate analysis of risk factors for coronary heart disease. Circulation 48:950–958.

Nutritional Factors in Hypertension
© 1990 Alan R. Liss, Inc., pages 51–65

4 Nutrition and Blood Pressure in Childhood

Bonita Falkner, M.D.
Andrew I. Rabinowitz, B.S.
Suzanne H. Michel, M.P.H., R.D.

INTRODUCTION

There is presently sufficient evidence to indicate that cardiovascular diseases, including hypertension and atherosclerosis, have their onset in the young [5,48,64,87]. The pathogenic processes which ultimately progress to vascular injury during adulthood are operational in childhood. Hypertension and atherosclerotic cardiovascular disease are disorders determined by a genetic constellation of predisposing physiologic elements [31]. Environmental factors including dietary patterns serve as precipitating factors inducing or enhancing the variant predisposing elements. Much remains to be done in dissecting and delineating these processes. A concurrent approach involves the development and application of preventative measures that may be applied at a young age.

Clinically, we are not yet able to identify the prehypertensive child. We may, however, approach a selection of potential future hypertensives by assessment of risk factors. It is this young "at risk" population who may benefit from early intervention. Nonpharmacologic approaches, such as dietary interventions in the treatment of hypertension, have recently received increased attention [40]. These dietary interventions may also have some rationale for application in the young. This chapter will discuss the issues of diet as preventative and therapeutic interventions in the young, including the

From the Department of Pediatrics, Hahnemann University, Broad and Vine Streets, Philadelphia, PA 19102.

areas of growth, obesity, sodium, and potassium. We will also discuss these interventions as they may relate to current dietary behaviors in children and the effectiveness, feasibility, and safety of using dietary modification for preventative treatments in the young.

BLOOD PRESSURE AND GROWTH

A relationship between blood pressure and growth has been demonstrated. Blood pressure increases as a child ages from birth through adolescence. This increase in blood pressure is not, however, uniform from individual to individual, nor is it continuous throughout childhood. Blood pressure increases from birth to six months of age. This initial increase is followed by a plateau phase spanning from 6 months to 15 months in some children, and to 24 months in others. During this time period, there is no increase in blood pressure, while the average child experiences a 16% increase in height and a 37% increase in weight [65]. A definite explanation for this period of growth without a concomitant increase in blood pressure has yet to be demonstrated. The plateau phase is succeeded by a slight increase in blood pressure lasting until the fifth year of life. Voors et al. found that after five or six years of age, blood pressure shows an accelerated rate of rise with age in children 5 to 14 years old [83]. Another study has shown a gradual yet continuous increase in the systolic as well as the diastolic component of blood pressure from 7 to 18 years of age [12]. In females, blood pressure seems to plateau at about 14 years of age [63]. In the young adult male, pressure reaches a plateau between the sixteenth and eighteenth years and no further rise is observed until age 21 [48].

The increase in blood pressure through adolescence, in males, can be attributed to the increases in height and body mass rather than to advancing age [4,57,82]. In a study that controlled for weight, height, and body mass, it was shown that body mass rather than age correlated with blood pressure in the decade from ages 5 to 14 [82]. Lauer found that the strongest relationships with blood pressure level and trend were with body weight level and trend, respectively. Children exhibiting the greatest upward trend in systolic blood pressure also demonstrated the greatest upward trends in body size measures [45]. This positive correlation between height, body mass, and basal blood pressure has also been demonstrated by several additional studies [36,47,49,57,82].

OBESITY

With the demonstration that body weight has a definite effect upon blood pressure, researchers have examined the possibility that excessive body weight might cause or accompany abnormally high levels of blood pressure. Obesity in adults was shown to be a significant risk factor for the development of essential hypertension [22]. Recent studies have attempted to investigate whether obesity at a particular stage of childhood causes or contributes to a transient or permanent hypertensive condition. Stamler found that in younger adults, overweight was associated with at least double the prevalence of diastolic hypertension [72]. Those who were near desirable weight initially and experienced little or no weight gain were at a smaller risk of hypertension than were those who as young adults were above desirable weight and had weight gain [70].

If obesity is thus taken to be a risk factor for the development of hypertension, then the origins of obesity must be examined. This question has been approached from epidemiological and sociological, as well as genetic, perspectives. It has been demonstrated that in the absence of parental obesity, the incidence of obesity in children was 14%; if one parent was obese, the incidence rose to 41%; and if both parents were obese, the incidence was 81% [56]. Such evidence indicates that obesity is an inherited trait that is polygenic [9].

Despite these findings, many have argued that obesity might not be inherited, but rather the result of a shared environment. Advocates of this line of thought propose that a child becomes obese by observing and ultimately adopting the eating habits of an obese parent or parents. Those who favor the genetic basis of obesity have attempted to substantiate their claims using twin studies.

It has been shown that monozygotic (MZ) twins were more concordant in body size when reared apart than were dizygotic (DZ) twins of the same sex [56,74]. When skinfold was used as a criterion, it was shown that the average difference in skinfold is three times greater in DZ twins than MZ twins. The distribution of skinfold measurements as compared to a normal distribution supports the theory that weight is a multifactorial or polygenic trait [9]. It cannot be stated that environment plays no role in obesity, but rather that environmental factors may enhance or dampen the effects of a genetic predisposition.

Researchers have also attempted to test the genetic theory for blood pressure by examining the relationship between blood pressures of mothers and their infants. There has been a small but significant aggregation of diastolic pressure of newborn and the corresponding diastolic pressure of the mother [47]. Zinner believes that each person's blood pressure is channelized reasonably early [88]. This channel is fixed at a young age. Thus, low pressures tend to remain low and high pressures tend to remain high [26]. Finally, for both systolic and diastolic pressures, variance of blood pressure scores were significantly less within families than among all children in a given age group

[88]. There is epidemiological evidence suggesting that a relationship does exist between the genetic determinant for body weight and for blood pressure.

Higher levels of blood pressure in childhood may be a predictor of future hypertension. If an obese child is allowed to remain obese, there is an added probability that the child may become hypertensive. Thus, the best approach to limiting adult essential hypertension would be through weight reduction in childhood. Attention to minimizing excessive weight gain at a particular period of life, such as in the young, might have long-term beneficial effects in preventing subsequent hypertension or excess blood pressure with aging [36]. The Muscatine Study showed that some children who lost weight also showed decreases in blood pressure [62]. Dustan demonstrated that weight reduction reduces arterial pressure in both normotensive and hypertensive persons [22]. Chiang et al. [13] referred to 14 studies in which dietary weight reduction without sodium restriction, in patients and volunteers, was accompanied by a decrease in blood pressure. Thus, it appears that weight reduction and maintenance instituted in youth may be a preventative measure to hypertension [22,36,39]. Perhaps the most convincing of the recent studies on weight reduction in children was conducted by Brownell. This study placed overweight children on a program that stressed both behavioral and dietary modification. Those children who had the highest pressures initially had the largest reductions in pressure during treatment, and these subjects were successful in maintaining losses. Utilizing this program, 80% of the subjects showed a significant decrease in systolic blood pressure and 70% showed decreases in diastolic pressure. Weight changes were highly correlated with changes in systolic blood pressure rather than with diastolic blood pressure [11].

The physiological basis for the effect of obesity on hypertension is not fully understood. However, childhood obesity predicts adult obesity, and hence added risk for cardiovascular disease. Therefore, the potential benefits of weight control are apparent. Such a program should be started in childhood, when prevention might prove most effective.

SODIUM

Many classic epidemiologic studies have described a correlation of the level of chronic dietary sodium intake among populations with the prevalence of hypertension [20,71]. These observations have resulted in the concept that sodium plays an etiologic role in the development of essential hypertension. Despite the experimental and population data, the association of sodium intake with blood pressure among individuals within a given population has been difficult to demonstrate [21,77]. Evidence elucidating a direct effect of sodium intake on blood pressure in children is even more sparse. Several studies have investigated the effect of sodium content in drinking water on blood pressure in children. These reports have yielded conflicting results [32,35,38,61,81].

Cooper et al. [16] were able to demonstrate a quantitatively weak but significant linear relationship between blood pressure and sodium excretion in children age 11 to 14 years. However, these observations required seven consecutive 24-hour urine collections per subject to adjust for intraindividual variation. The variability of blood pressure, dietary sodium intake, and sodium excretion in childhood all render a significant correlation of sodium intake with blood pressure difficult to identify, if indeed one does exist. Hofman et al. [38] performed a randomized, controlled sodium intake trial on infants. These investigators compared blood pressure in infants receiving a low-sodium formula to those receiving usual formula. A small but statistically significant difference in blood pressure was found at 6 months of life with infants fed the lower-sodium formula having a lower blood pressure.

In established hypertension, a reduction in dietary sodium may reduce blood pressure [52]. Dietary maneuvers to lower sodium intake may also lower blood pressure in normotensive young adults [19]. Data on the effects of reduced sodium on blood pressure in children are limited and at this time equivocal. Cooper and associates studied the effect of dietary sodium restriction on blood pressure in adolescents, using a randomized crossover trial design. Following 24 days of sodium restriction, there was no effect on blood pressure in these normotensive adolescents [17]. The effect of sodium restriction on blood pressure in offspring of normotensive and hypertensive parents was investigated by Watt et al. Their subjects were adolescents and young adults (mean age 22 years). Sodium intake was reduced for 8 weeks in a double-blind, placebo-controlled randomized crossover trial on 66 subjects. The investigators found no significant difference in blood pressure in children with and without parental hypertension following the low-sodium intervention. [85] On the other hand, Falkner et al. [25] studied adolescents with and without parental hypertension by sodium loading. Normotensive adolescents were loaded with 10 gm NaCl daily in addition to their usual diet for 14 days. Some offspring of hypertensive parents had a significant increase in blood pressure, indicating that they were sensitive to sodium. Offspring of normotensive parents had no change in blood pressure, indicating that they were resistant to the high-sodium intake.

In both man and experimental animals, the blood pressure response to sodium intake varies. This has resulted in the concept of sodium sensitivity or sodium resistance. Although the definition of sodium sensitivity varies according to different investigators, the concept implies an increased blood pressure response to sodium loading or decreased blood pressure response to sodium depletion. Weinberger and associates have performed extensive studies on sodium sensitivity in adults and have reported a greater prevalence of sodium sensitivity in blacks and with increasing age [86]. Studies of sodium sensitivity in children are limited. In addition to the above-noted study of sodium loading on normotensive adolescents [25], we have also performed sodium-loading studies on young adults (18–22 years). With our chronic oral loading protocol, we have found different prevalence rates of sodium sensitivity by race with 22% of whites and 53% of blacks demonstrating a sodium-sensitive response [24].

The identification of a young individual who is sensitive to sodium intake on the basis of blood pressure response does provide a more rational basis on which to implement specific dietary maneuvers. However, the means of identification, at present, are extremely arduous and not practical to apply to normal populations of children or adults. Furthermore, it is unlikely that sodium operates as an isolated etiologic factor. Other investigations have pursued the interaction of sodium intake with other physiologic parameters. Several studies have demonstrated an interrelationship between neurogenic activity and sodium intake [50,55,76]. Luft et al. [51] have shown a decrease in sympathetic activity with increasing sodium load. The effect of a higher sodium intake on sodium-sensitive or sodium-resistant individuals appears to depend on a relationship between total blood volume and vascular resistance. In normal subjects, the forearm blood flow increases and forearm vascular resistance decreases [42]. In borderline hypertension, the reverse occurs with increasing sodium intake [53]. Sullivan et al. have demonstrated that sodium-sensitive young adults also have a decrease in forearm blood flow and an increase in resistance with a higher sodium intake [75]. The results of these investigations suggest that a sodium-sensitive blood pressure response is related to adrenergic activity and to vascular tone. It is possible that in childhood a high sodium intake modulates the activity of these interrelationships. However, the effect on the measurement of pressure may not be perceived for several years. Further studies will be necessary to clarify these questions.

POTASSIUM

There has been a recent resurgence of interest in the level of dietary potassium as a factor in hypertension. Studies on primitive populations indicate an inverse relationship between potassium intake and blood pressure. Other studies indicate that a reduction in the dietary sodium-to-potassium ratio reduces blood pressure [80]. Experimental studies in rats [79] and dogs [1,2] have shown a beneficial effect of potassium on preventing vascular lesions and lowering blood pressure.

Watson and associates studied urinary sodium-to-potassium ratio in black and white adolescent females. They found a significant correlation between the ratio of sodium:potassium excreted and diastolic blood pressure. Additionally, this ratio was significantly higher in the black females than in the white females [84]. It has been suggested by Corrigan and Langford [18] that a lower dietary potassium intake may account for the greater incidence of hypertension among blacks in the United States.

Berenson et al. [5] also found a lower urinary potassium excretion in black children. They also demonstrated that in response to oral potassium (80 mEq/day) there was a natriuresis and a reduction in blood pressure. The observation by Sullivan et al. [76] of higher serum and urinary potassium levels in young individuals with borderline hypertension resistant to dietary sodium load suggested that potassium blunted the effect of the high sodium intake [76]. In another related study, Skrabal et al. [69] studied the effect of a low sodium/high potassium diet on 20 young normotensive adults, 10 of whom had a family history of hypertension. This diet reduced the diastolic blood pressure by an average of 5 mmHg in 10 of 20 subjects, of whom 7 had a family history of hypertension. In all subjects, the low sodium/high potassium diet reduced the blood pressure rise produced by norepinephrine infusion, or by mental stress [69].

These studies indicate that potassium, which has a natriuretic effect, can modify the activity of the central and peripheral nervous system. In addition, potassium may alter the renin-angiotensin system, as well as affect vascular tone [80]. The role of dietary potassium on Na/K ratio as a regulator of blood pressure in the young requires further investigation. However, at present, there exists sufficient evidence to encourage a higher dietary potassium intake in children who are at risk for hypertension.

In addition to sodium and potassium, other ions may contribute significantly to blood pressure regulation. Blaustein hypothesized that a sodium/calcium exchange mechanism is one of the mechanisms controlling intracellular calcium activity, and as such, controls vascular tone [7]. Several population surveys and brief intervention studies report results that are variable in the association of calcium intake with blood pressure [3,15,34,73]. While it is plausible that calcium may play a significant role in blood pressure regulation, further study is necessary to clarify this role.

CURRENT DIET PATTERNS

While the scientific debate regarding diet and hypertension continues, the need to advise parents and formulate policy statements regarding diet and hypertension is ever present. Recent nutrition policy statements from the U.S. government have recommended a reduced intake of dietary sodium for the general population [33]. These recommendations are based not only on research linking sodium to hypertension, but also on evidence that the sodium content of the typical North American's diet is increasing [8]. The average American diet contains 4 to 7 grams of sodium. In the past, equal amounts of sodium were derived from naturally occurring sodium in food, salt used in food processing, and table salt. Current surveys indicate that 1/6 of dietary sodium is from that naturally occurrs in food, 1/3 from table salt, and 1/2 from sodium in processed foods [8]. The increased use of processed foods and decreased use of natural foods that are very low in sodium and high in potassium content reverses this ratio and has altered the usual sodium: potassium content of the American diet. Although some companies have recently attempted to reduce the sodium content of their products [27], processed and fabricated foods continue to contribute a significant portion of sodium to the diet. In addition, family eating styles have shifted toward an increased use of processed foods and restaurant meals.

Attention to the sodium content of the diet begins in infancy. Prior to 1920, the majority of infants were fed human milk and the introduction of table foods was withheld until after the first birthday. Average sodium intake was 5 to 10 mEq per day. During the 1960s and early 1970s, sodium intake rose to 41 mEq per day, well above the current recommendation of 5 to 15 mEq/day. Laughlin has noted a steady increase in the amount of sodium in infant diets up to 1977 due to the introduction, in this country, of milk-based formulas and commercially prepared infant foods [46]. In response to both consumer and professional concerns, formula companies reduced the amount of sodium in their preparations and infant-food manufacturers reduced and subsequently removed all added salt from their products. Of great concern were reports of the high sodium content of some homemade infant foods [41].

Parents who make their own infant foods should be instructed to avoid adding salt to the baby food in order to satisfy their own taste preference. Current average sodium intake for infants under six months of age is 30.7 mEq per day [68].

Although the total amount of sodium in infant diets has declined with the recent reduction of sodium in formulas and commercially prepared baby foods, surveys indicate the acutal amount of sodium consumed by infants over six months of age remains above the levels recommended by the American Academy of Pediatrics and the RDA. The major contributing factor to the elevated intake is the use of cow's milk and table foods in the second six months of life [54,58]. The use of cow's milk along with a balanced diet during this time period has been advocated by the American Academy of Pediatrics [28]. Schaefer et al. [66] studied maternal behavior and infant feeding practices as related to salt use. The results indicated that maternal education had the greatest influence on infant feeding habits and sodium use. Addition of salt to infant foods was predicted by maternal salt use and by positive family history of hypertension [66]. The findings of increased sodium intake during the second half of the first year of life and the results of Schaefer's study speak of the need for comprehensive infant-feeding guidance for families at high risk for the development of hypertension.

The young child is dependent upon the family to provide nourishment. This relationship influences the child's food habits, and when choices are not appropriate may contribute to the development of nutrition-related chronic diseases. A child's food choices may also be influenced by the media. By the late teens, the average child has watched fifteen thousand hours of television. During that time, they have been prompted to buy numerous items, including cereals, snack foods, and meals at fast-food restaurants. Many of these foods contain large amounts of sodium and contribute to excessive sodium intake. Parents need appropriate guidance in their attempts to combat the influence of the media in order to provide an appropriate diet for their children. Regional surveys have shown an increased use of snacks as a major source of the child's nutrient intake. With this intake pattern, the food choices result in a diet that is high in fat, salt, or sugar. National surveys note the average daily sodium intake for the young child is 78.5 mEq or 185% of the RDA. The major food source of sodium in this age range is grain and cereal products [68].

The typical adolescent consumes 291 mEg of sodium per day, which is 203% of the RDS [68]. Surveys have indicated that the adolescent consumes more fat, added sugar, protein, and sodium than is currently advised [23]. A substantial portion of their intake may be consumed as snacks that are obtained in the form of processed convenience foods in the home or from food purchased from vendors, fast-food restaurants, vending machines, or school feeding programs. As family structure changes, teenagers become more responsible for the preparation of their own meals. The teen years are times for experimentation, and it is during this time that alternative eating styles may be attempted. Boulton [10] has reviewed the unique nutritional challenges presented by the adolescent and possible methods of altering nutrient intake.

The need for dietary intervention in the pediatric age range for control of hypertension in latter life is obvious. Several European countries have instituted national programs for hypertension control. Norway has designed a program that addresses the issue of dietary change through efforts to alter individual habits and knowledge. This program also regulates, on a national level, the availability of appropriate foods. Australia has developed a school-based health and nutrition program, and England has published

"New British Diet" with strategies for implementation [10]. Although the United States does not have a national nutrition program for the control of hypertension, national policies and goals have been issued that address the problem [33,59,78]. Recent FDA legislation requires manufacturers to meet specific guidelines if they make claims regarding the sodium content of their product. Professional and consumer organizations are recommending the removal of salt from the list of food additives defined as "generally regarded as safe" (GRAS) [67]. Federal food programs, such as the School Breakfast and Lunch Programs, should meet national nutrition goals by lowering the sodium content of their meals. On a more local level, in response to the USDA request to reduce the sodium content of school lunches, an individual school district has modified the sodium content of recipes, with positive results [30].

Individual institutions and researchers in the United States have designed and implemented intervention programs for adults, but few programs have focused on the needs of the pediatric population. Farris et al.[25a] reviewed methodology used to assess the nutrition education needs of teenagers relative to cardiovascular diseases [25a]. Frank et al. have surveyed the usual nutrient intake and food habits of children and designed a primary hypertension prevention program for children [29]. The effectiveness of these programs needs to be demonstrated.

A national hypertension control program such as Norway's may not be feasible in this country because of a variety of eating styles and food habits. But there are mechanisms by which action can be taken to improve the nutrition status of the general population. Examples of such actions include: the expansion of the nutrition education component of federally funded food programs such as WIC and food stamps; school nutrition and health education programs initiated in the primary grades; the cooperation of industry in the reduction of sodium in processed foods; and the development of programs in the health-care system for effective screening, treatment, and follow-up in the pediatric population. Blackburn has discussed the need for education, persuasion, and legislation to bring about positive [8] environmental-behavioral factors that would lead to the reduction and prevention of hypertension in this country. Kumanyika and Bonner [43] have also described a social change–oriented community-based hypertension control program designed to meet the needs of black Americans.

A great deal of discussion surrounds the issue of sodium reduction. However, little has been said about the possible adverse effects of such a widespread policy. For example, children with cystic fibrosis have an increased sodium requirement; recent reports describe the complication of sodium depletion subsequent to the removal of salt from infant foods [46]. There is also concern that removal of iodized salt from the diet may lead to the resurgence of goiter [44]. In addition, the effect of a low sodium on consumption of other major nutrients, such as calcium and iron, needs to evaluated. Overall, the sodium intake of children is excessive. Due to shifting dietary patterns, the sodium intake of children may be rising. Therefore, a moderate reduction in the excessive sodium content of foods consumed by children would be safe and likely to provide some overall benefit to present and future health status of the young.

SUMMARY

The concept that primary prevention or modification of hypertension may be feasible through changes in diet is an attractive approach. There is evidence that modification of dietary intake of sodium and potassium may alter blood pressure levels in some individuals. However, more evidence needs to be developed along the line of precise identification of those who would be diet responders. At present, much can reasonably be done to recognize and modify risk for hypertension at a young age. These measures include control of childhood obesity as well as modification of diet patterns in at risk families to lower sodium and raise potassium intake. As more is delineated regarding the mechanism of hypertension, nutrition as therapy may become more specifically designed.

ACKNOWLEDGMENTS

Supported in part by a grant from NHLBI R01 HL 31802.

REFERENCES

1. Anderson DE, Kearns WD, Better WE (1983): Progressive hypertension in dogs by avoidance conditioning and saline infusion. Hypertension 5:286–291.
2. Anderson DE, Kearns WD, Worden TJ (1983): Potassium infusion attenuates avoidance-saline hypertension in dogs. Hypertension 5:415–420.
3. Belizan JM, Vilar J, Pineda O, Gonzalez AE, Sainz E, Garrera G, Sibrian R (1983): Reduction of blood pressure with calcium supplementation in young adults. JAMA 249: 1161–1165.
4. Berenson GS (1980): "Cardiovascular Risk Factors in Children." New York, Oxford: Oxford University Press. Andrews C, Hester H (eds.) pp 274–286.
5. Berenson GS, Cresanta JL, Weber LS (1984a): High blood pressure in the young. Ann Rev Med 35:535–560.
6. Berenson GS, Weber LS, Srinivasan SR, Cresanta JL, Frank GC, Farris R (1984b): Black-white contrasts as determinants of cardiovascular risk in childhood. Precursors of coronary artery and primary hypertensive diseases. Am Heart J 108:672–683.
7. Blaustein M (1977): Sodium ions, calcium ions, blood pressure regulation, and hypertension, a reassessment and a hypothesis. Am J Physiol 232 (1):c165.

8. Blackburn H, Prineas, R (1983): Diet and hypertension: Anthropology, epidemiology, and public health implications program. Biochem Pharmacol 19:31–79.
9. Borjeson M (1976): The aetiology of obesity in children. Acts Paedist Scandinav 65: 279–287.
10. Boulton, TJC (1985): Patterns of food intake in childhood and adolescence and risk of later disease or "The Awful Food Kids Eat Nowadays Must Be Bad For Them." Aust. Nz J Med 15:478–488.
11. Brownell KD, Kelmen JH, Stunkard AJ (1983): Treatment of obese children with and without their mothers: Changes in weight and blood pressure. Pediatrics, 71:515–523.
12. Cassimos G, Varlamis S, Karamperis S, Katsouyannopoulos V (1977): Blood pressure in children and adolescents. Acta Paed Scand 66:439–443.
13. Chiang BN, Perlman LV, Epstein FH (1969): Overweight and hypertension: A Review. Circulation 39:403.
14. Committee on Nutrition, American Academy of Pediatrics (1974): Salt intake and eating patterns of infants and children in relation to blood pressure. Pediatrics 53:115.
15. Connor SL, Connor WE, Henry H, Sexton G, Keenan EJ (1984): The effects of familial relationships, age, body weight and diet on blood pressure and the 24-hour urinary excretion of sodium, potassium and creatinine in men, women, and children of randomly selected families. Circulation 70:76–85.
16. Cooper R, Soltero I, Liu K, Berkson D, Levinson S, Stamler J (1980): The association between urinary sodium excretion and blood pressure in children. Circulation 62:97–104.
17. Cooper R, Van Horn L, Liu K (1984): A randomized trial on the effect of decreased dietary sodium intake on blood pressure in adolescents. J Hypertension 2:361–366.
18. Corrigan SA, Langford HG (1987): Dietary management of hypertension. Comprehensive Therapy 13:62–67.
19. Costa FV, Ambrosioni E, Montebugnoli L, Paccaloni L, Basconi L, Magnani B (1981): Effect of a low salt diet and of acute salt loading and blood pressure and intralymphocytic sodium concentration in young subjects with borderline hypertension. Clin Sci 51:21–23.
20. Dahl LK (1957): Evidence for an increase intake of sodium in hypertension based on urinary excretion of sodium. Proc Soc Exp Biol Med 94:23.
21. Dawber TR, Kannel WB, Kogan A, Donabedian RK, McNamara PR, Pearson G (1967): Environmental factors in hypertension: In Stamler J, Stamler R, Pullman TN (eds): "The Epidemiology of Hypertension." New York: Grave and Stratton, p 255.
22. Dustan HP (1983): Mechanisms of hypertension associated with obesity. Ann Intern Med 98 (pt 2):860–864.
23. Dwyer JP (1980): Diets for children and adolescents that meet the dietary goals. Am J Dis Child 134:1073.
24. Falkner B, Kushner H, Khalsa D, Canessa M, Katz S (1986): Sodium sensitivity, growth and family history of hypertension in young blacks. J Hypertension 4(suppl 5):S381–S383.
25. Falkner B, Onesti G, Angelakos E (1981): Effect of salt loading on the cardiovascular response to stress in adolescents. Hypertension 3:(suppl II):195–199.
25a. Farris RP, Cresanta JL, Croft JB, Webber LS, Frank GC, Berenson GS (1986): Macronutrient intakes of 10-yr-old children, 1973 to 1982. J Am Diet Assoc 86(6):765–770.
26. Feinleib M, Gordon T, Garrison RJ, (1969): Blood pressure and age: The Framingham Study. Presented at the Second Annual Meeting of the Society for Epidemiological Research, Chapel Hill, NC.
27. Filer LJ, JR. (1980): Appropriate consumption of sodium and potassium. In White PL, Crocco SC (ed): Sodium and potassium in foods and drugs. AM Med Assoc pp 8–16.
28. Fomon S, Filer LJ, Anderson TA, Ziegler E (1979): Recommendations for feeding normal infants. Pediatrics 63(1):52–59.

29. Frank GC, Gonzalez AE, Sainz E, Garrera G, Sibrian R (1982): An approach to primary preventive treatment for children with high blood pressure in a total community. J Am Col Nutr 1(4):357–374.
30. Frank GC, White M (1983): Application of a sodium-modified recipe program in school lunch. Sch. Foodserv. Res. Rev, Denver: American School Food Service Association, vol. 7, issue 2, pp 112–114.
31. Folkow B (1982): Physiological aspects of primary hypertension. Physiol Rev 62:347.
32. Folson AR, Prineas RJ (1982): Drinking water composition and blood pressure: A review of the epidemiology. Am J Epidemiol 115:818–832.
33. Food and Nutrition Board, National Research Council: Toward Healthful Diets (1980). Washington, D.C.: National Academy of Sciences.
34. Garcia-Palmieri MR, Costas R, Cruz-Vidal M, Sorlie PD, Tillotson J, Havlik R (1984): Milk consumption, calcium intake and decreased hypertension in Puerto Rico. Hypertension 6:322–328.
35. Hallenback WH, Brenninmon GR, Anderson RJ (1981): High sodium in drinking water and its effect on blood pressure. Am J Epidemiol 114:817–826.
36. Havlick RJ, Hubert HB, Fabsitz RR, Feinleib M (1983): Weight and hypertension. Ann Intern Med 98 (pt 2):855–859.
37. Hofman A, Hazelbrock A, Valkenburg HA (1983): A randomized trial of sodium intake and blood pressure in newborn infants. JAMA 250:370–373.
38. Hofman A, Valhenburg HA, Vaandroger GJ (1980): Increased blood pressure in school children related to high sodium levels of drinking water. J Epidemiol Commun Health 34:179–181.
39. Johnson AL, Carnoni JC, Cassel JC, Tyroler HA, Heyden S, Hames CG (1975): Influence of race, sex, and weight on blood pressure behavior in young adults. Am J Cardiol 35:523–530.
40. Joint Committee on the Detection, Evaluation, and Treatment of High Blood Pressure: The 1984 Report of the Joint National Committee on detection, evaluation, and treatment of high blood pressure. Arch Intern Med 144:1045–1057.
41. Kerr M, Reisinger KS, Plankey FW (1978): Sodium concentration of homemade baby foods. Pediatrics 62(3):331–335.
42. Kukendall WM, Connor WE, Abboud F, Rastogi SP, Anderson TA, Fry M (1972): The effect of dietary sodium on blood pressure of normotensive men. In Genesti J (ed): "International Symposium on Renin-Angiotension: Adolescence-Sodium in hypertension." Berlin: Springer-Verlag, pp 360–373.
43. Kumanyika S, Bonner M (1985): Toward a lower-sodium lifestyle in black communities. J Natl Med Assoc 77:969–975.
44. Krause MV, Mahan KL (1984): "Food, Nutrition, and Diet Therapy". Philadelphia: W.B. Saunders Company, ch. 28, p 558.
45. Lauer RM, Clarke WR, Beaglehole R (1984): Level, trend, and variability of blood pressure during childhood: The Muscatine Study. Circulation 69(2):242–249.
46. Laughlin J, Brady MS, Eigen H (1981): Changing feeding trends as a cause of electrolyte depletion in infants with cystic fibrosis. Pediatrics 68(2):203–207.
47. Lee Y-H, Rosner B, Courld JB, Lowe EW, Kass EH (1976): Familial aggregation of blood pressures of newborn infants and their mothers. Pediatrics 58:722–729.
48. Londe S, Bourgoignie JJ, Robson AM, Goldring D (1971): Hypertension in apparently normal children. J Peds 78:569.
49. Londe S, Goldring D (1972): Hypertension in children. Am Heart J 84:1–4.
50. Luft FC, Grim CE, Higgins JT Jr, Weinberger MH (1977): Difference in response to sodium administration in normotensive white and black subjects. J Lab Clin Med 90:555–562.

51. Luft FC, Rankin LI, Henry DP, Bloch R, Grim CE, Weyman AE, Murray RH, Weinberger MH: (1979): Plasma and urinary norepinephrine values at extreme of sodium intake in normal men. Hypertension 1:261.
52. Macgregor GA, Best F, Cam J (1982): Double-blind randomized crossover trial of moderate sodium restriction in essential hypertension. Lancet 1:351–355.
53. Mark AL, Lawton J, Abboud FM, Fitz AE, Connor WE, Heistad DD (1975): Effects of high and low sodium intake on arterial pressure and forearm vascular resistance in borderline hypertension. Circulation 36 (suppl I):194.
54. Martinez GA, Ryan AS, Malec DJ (1985): Nutrient intakes of American infants and children fed cow's milk or infant formulas. AJDC 139:1010–1018.
55. Masuo K, Ogihara T, Kumahara Y, Yamatodani A, Wada H (1984): Increased plasma norepinephrine in young patients with essential hypertension under three sodium intakes. Hypertension 6:315–321.
56. Mayer J (1975): Obesity during childhood. In Winick M (ed): "Current Concepts in Nutrition. Vol. 3. Childhood Obesity." New York: Wiley, pp 6.
57. Miall WE, Lovell HG (1967): Relation between change of blood pressures and age. Br Med J 2:660.
58. Montalto B, Berenson JD, Martinez GA (1985): Nutrient intakes of formula-fed infants and infants fed cow's milk. Pediatrics 75(2):343–351.
59. Nutrition and Your Health. Dietary Guidelines for Americans (1980). Home and Garden Bulletin No. 232. Washington, D.C.; U.S. Dept. of Agriculture, U.S. Dept. of Health and Human Services.
61. Pomrehn PR, Clarke WR, Sowers MF, Wallace RB, Lauer RM (1983): Community differences in blood pressure levels and drinking water sodium. Am J Epidemiol 118: 60–71.
62. Rames LK, Clarke WR, Connor WE, Reiter MA, Lauer RM (1978): Normal blood pressures and the evaluation of sustained blood pressure evaluation in childhood: The Muscatine Study. Pediatrics 61:245–251.
63. Report of the Second Task Force on Blood Pressure Control in Children—1987. Pediatrics 79:1–25.
64. Report of the Task Force on Blood Pressure Control in Children. Peds 58 (suppl):797.
65. Schacter J, Kuller LH, Perfetti C (1982): Blood pressure during the first two years of life. Am J Epidemiol 116:29–41.
66. Schaefer L, Kumanyika SK (1985): Maternal variables related to potentially high-sodium infant feeding practices. J AM Dietet Assoc 85:433–438.
67. Select Committee on GRAS Substances (1979): Evaluation of the health aspects of sodium chloride as a food ingredient. Life Science Research Office, Fed. Am. Society of Experimental Biology.
68. Shank F.R., Park YK, Harland BF, Vanderveen JE, Forbers AL, Prosky L (1982): Perspective of food and drug administration of dietary sodium. J. Am. Diet. Assoc. 80:29.
69. Skrabal F, Aubock J, Hortnagi H (1981): Low sodium-high potassium diet for prevention of hypertension. Protable mechanisms of action. Lancet Oct:885–900.
70. Stamler J: "Epidemiology of hypertension" (1967): New York: Grune and Stratton, pp 104–108.
71. Stamler J, Katz LN, Pick R, Rodbard S (1955): Dietary and hormonal factors in experimental atherogenesis and blood pressure regulation. In Pincus G. (ed): "Recent Progress in Hormone Research." New York: Academic Press, pp 401–452.
72. Stamler R, Stamler J, Reidinger W (1978): Weight and blood pressure, findings in hypertension screening of 1 million Americans. J Am Med Assoc 240 no. 15.
73. Stanton JL, Braitman LE, Riley AM, Koo CS, Smith JL (1982): Demographic, dietary,

life style and anthropometric correlates of blood pressure. Hypertension 4 (suppl III): 136–142.

74. Stunkard AJ (1980): Obesity. Phila: W.B. Saunders Co. pp 48–54.
75. Sullivan JM, Prewitt RL, Ratts TE, Josephs JA, Connor MJ (1987): Hemodynamic characteristics of sodium-sentitive human subjects. Hypertension 9:398–406.
76. Sullivan JM, Ratts TE, Taylor JC, Kraus DH, Barton BR, Patrick DR, Reed SW (1980): Hemodynamic effects of dietary sodium in man. Hypertension 2:506.
77. Swaye PS, Girrord, RW, Berrenttoni JN (1972): Dietary salt and essential hypertension. Am J Cardiol 29:33.
78. The Surgeon General's Report on Health (1979): "Healthy People." Report on Health Promotion, and Disease Prevention. Public Health Service. Washington, D.C.: U.S. Government Printing Office.
79. Tobin L, MacNeil D, Johnson MA, Ganguli MC, Iwaj J (1984): Potassium protection against lesions of the renal tubules, arteries, and glomeruli and nephron loss in salt-loaded hypertensive Dahl S. rats. Hypertension 6:(suppl I):170–176.
80. Treasure J, Ploth D (1983): Role of dietary potassium in the treatment of hypertension. Hypertension 5:864–872.
81. Tuthill RW and Calabrese EJ (1979): Elevated sodium levels in the public drinking water as a contributor to elevated blood pressure levels in the community. Arch Environ Health 34:194–204.
82. Voors AW, Webber LS, Frerichs RR (1977): Body, height, and body mass as determinants of basal blood pressure in the Bogalusa Study. Am J Epidemiol 106:101.
83. Voors, SW, Foster TA, Freriches RR, Webber LS, Berenson G (1976): The Bogalusa Heart Study. Circulation 54:319–327.
84. Watson RL, Langford HG, Aberneth J, (1980): Urinary electrolytes, body weight, and blood pressure, pooled cross- sectional results among four groups of adolescent females. Hypertension 2 (suppl 1):193–198.
85. Walt GCM, Edward SC, Hart JT, Hart M, Walton P, Foy CJW (1983): Dietary sodium and arterial blood pressure: Evidence against genetic susceptibility. Br Med J 286: 432–435.
86. Weinberger MH, Miller JZ, Luft FC, Grim CE, Fineberg NS (1968): Definitions and characteristics of sodium sensitivity and blood pressure resistance. Hypertension 8 (suppl II):127–134.
87. Zinner SA, Levy PS, Kass EH (1971a): Family aggregation of blood pressure in childhood. N Engl J Med 283:461.
88. Zinner SH, Levy PS, Kass EH (1971b): Familial aggregation of blood pressure in childhood. N Engl J Med 284:(8):401–404.

Nutritional Factors in Hypertension
© *1990 Alan R. Liss, Inc., pages 67–77*

5	# Relationship of Body Fat Distribution to Blood Pressure Level
	Linda M. Gerber, Ph.D.

INTRODUCTION

The association between obesity and hypertension in populations has been recognized for many years. Hypertension is more prevalent among obese populations [1], and there is an increased prevalence of obesity among hypertensive subjects [2]. The causal relationship, however, of obesity and hypertension has not been established. The majority of obese individuals are not hypertensive, and several studies support the existence of confounding variables in the association of fatness and blood pressure [3–5].

Recent studies have shown that obesity is not a single entity and that the anatomic location of fat tissue plays an important role in predicting metabolic and blood pressure abnormalities [6–9]. Vague [10], as early as 1956, proposed that characterizing obesity based on the distribution of adipose tissue related to metabolic complications. Obesity with a fat distribution characteristic of men ("android" or upper-body obesity) was more closely associated with diabetes, gout, and atherosclerosis than the more peripheral distribution characteristic of women ("gynoid" or lower-body obesity).

While Vague was the first to quantify observations that upper-body obesity was associated with disorders of carbohydrate and lipid metabolism, the sex difference in the distribution of body fat was noted much earlier. As discussed by Stern and Haffner [11] in their review of body fat distribution

From the Cardiovascular Center, Cornell University Medical College, 525 East 68th Street, Starr 4, New York, NY 10021.

and hyperinsulinemia as risk factors for diabetes and cardiovascular disease, Rodin's statue of Balzac indicates that the sculptor viewed the typical male as having a powerful upper body and prominent abdomen. Furthermore, prehistoric cave art of "Venus figures" illustrates the association of female fertility with lower-body obesity.

Recent studies have confirmed Vague's observations [6,7] and have indicated that the distribution of fat deposits may be related to diabetes [12,13] and coronary heart disease [14,15]. One study related the distribution of body fat to the development of hyperglycemia among hypertensive men [16]. Fewer studies examine the relationship between hypertension and body fat distribution. This paper will review both cross-sectional and prospective studies among adults paying particular attention to the role of body fat distribution as an independent contributor to the development of hypertension.

MEASURES OF BODY FAT DISTRIBUTION

Various measures attempting to quantify body fat and its distribution have been used, including skinfold thickness, circumference, intra-abdominal, and subcutaneous abdominal fat measurements. Skinfold thickness has been measured primarily at the following sites: subscapular, triceps, and abdomen. A high subscapular-to-triceps skinfold ratio has been used as a measure of central as opposed to a more peripheral distribution of body fat [3,17]. Other investigators have used principal-component analysis [18,19] to reduce multiple measurements of skinfold thicknesses to fewer independent factors aiding the explanation of relationships.

Circumferences at the waist, arm, chest, thigh, and hips have also been used in describing body fat patterns. The waist-to-hip circumference ratio has recently been used as an index to categorize individuals as predominantly upper- or lower-body obese [6,8,20].

In contrast to measurements of skinfold thickness at specific sites and measurements of body circumferences, computed tomography measures fat in internal body compartments. Intra-abdominal fat can now be measured and subcutaneous fat can be quantified more accurately using this technique [21–23]. The ratio of intra-abdominal-to-subcutaneous abdominal fat has been found to be higher in individuals with predominantly upper-body obesity than in those with predominantly lower-body obesity [22].

CROSS-SECTIONAL STUDIES

A number of cross-sectional studies have reported an association between body fat distribution and blood pressure [3,7,8,9,17,24]. These studies have included men and women, blacks and whites, and obese and nonobese (see

TABLE 1. Cross-sectional Studies of Body Fat Distribution and Blood Pressure

Author (reference)	Number of subjects	Measure of body fat distribution
Hartz et al. [8]	21,065 women	Waist-to-hip ratio
Blair et al. [17]	2,051 men	Subscapular skinfold
	3,589 women	Triceps skinfold
Krotkiewski et al. [7]	253 women	Waist-to-hip ratio
Weinsier et al. [3]	87 men	Arm-to-thigh ratio
	312 women	Subscapular-to-triceps ratio
Kalkhoff et al. [9]	110 women	Waist-to-hip ratio
Seidell et al. [24]	95 men	Waist-to-hip ratio
	210 women	Waist-to-thigh ratio

Table 1). Various measures of body fat distribution were used, and, in all cases, a positive relation was found between centrally located or upper-body fat predominance and blood pressure.

In the study by Hartz et al. [8], hypertension was ascertained by a self-reported questionnaire for 21,065 nonobese and obese women. Waist and hip circumferences were self-measured and a ratio of waist-to-hip circumference was derived. Although a strong association between relative weight and hypertension was found, the waist-to-hip ratio was significantly related to hypertension even after adjusting for relative weight. Additionally, the prevalence of hypertension was approximately 26% in women with a waist-to-hip ratio less than 0.72 compared to 49% in women with a ratio greater than 0.81.

In the Health and Nutrition Examination Survey (HANES-1), subscapular skinfold had greater predictive power for both systolic and diastolic blood pressure than triceps skinfold [17]. The finding that blood pressure is associated more directly with centrally than peripherally deposited body fat held for both sexes and races.

Krotkiewski et al. compared blood pressures of obese women who had waist-to-hip circumference ratios either above or below average [7]. They found that the group with the higher ratio also had higher levels of both systolic and diastolic blood pressures in most of the body fat classes.

Using two measures of body fat distribution, an upper-body fat pattern— defined by an arm-to-thigh circumference ratio, and a central-body fat pattern—defined by a subscapular-to-triceps skinfold ratio, Weinsier et al. examined the contribution of fat pattern to blood pressure level [3]. Of the two indices, the upper-body fat pattern was found to be more highly predictive of blood pressure level. In addition to distribution of body fat, the following parameters combined explained 37% of the variation of mean arterial pressure: lean body mass, age, body build, and family history of hypertension. As a result, the authors concluded that the association between weight and blood pressure may be due to age or some aspect of body composition other than fatness *per se* [3].

In 110 obese, healthy women, Kalkhoff et al. [9] examined the relationship of body fat distribution, defined by the waist-to-hip ratio, to blood pressure. They found positive, significant correlations between the waist-to-hip ratio and both systolic and diastolic blood pressures. Furthermore, when these women were retrospectively segregated into the upper 25% of the waist-to-hip ratio range and the lowest 25% of this range, average blood pressures were found to differ substantially. Although within normal levels, both systolic and diastolic pressures were significantly higher among women with body fat accumulated predominantly on the upper body. The mean systolic blood pressure was 136 mmHg compared to 125 mmHg (p < 0.05) among upper- and lower-body obese women, respectively, while mean diastolic blood pressure was 84 mmHg compared to 76 mmHg (p < 0.01).

Seidell et al. [24] measured circumference of the waist, hip, and thigh and calculated the ratios of the waist-to-hip and waist-to-thigh in 95 men and 210 women. These ratios were linked to retrospective morbidity data; diagnoses made by general practitioners during the previous 17 years were included in the morbidity analysis. These investigators found a strong association between hypertension and a high waist-to-hip ratio for men, and a more moderate association between hypertension and a high waist-to-thigh ratio for both men and women. The results confirm that fat distribution, as measured by circumference ratios, is associated with the prevalence of hypertension, at least retrospectively reported.

PROSPECTIVE STUDIES

Numerous cross-sectional studies have shown an association between body fat distribution and hypertension; however, prospective studies are needed to demonstrate whether the distribution of body fat is important for the development of hypertension. A review of the literature yields no such prospective studies among adults, although four studies [14,15,19,25] report on the role of fat patterning as a risk factor for cardiovascular disease (see Table 2).

In a follow-up study of women in Gothenburg, Sweden, Lapidus et al. [14] found a significant positive relationship between the waist-to-hip ratio and the 12-year incidence of myocardial infarction, angina pectoris, stroke, and total mortality. Although general indices of obesity such as body mass index or sum of skinfold thicknesses predicted myocardial infarction, the waist-to-hip ratio seemed to be a stronger and more consistent predictor.

TABLE 2. Prospective Studies of Body Fat Distribution and Cardiovascular Disease

Author (reference)	Number of subjects	Length of follow-up	Measure of body fat distribution
Lapidus et al. [14]	1,462 women	12 years	Waist-to-hip ratio
Larsson et al. [15]	792 men	13 years	Waist-to-hip ratio
Ducimetiere et al. [19]	6,718 men	6.6 years	13 skinfolds
Stokes et al. [25]	1,934 men	22 years	4 skinfolds
	2,420 women		Waist circumference

Furthermore, unlike body-mass index and sum of skinfold thicknesses, the ratio also predicted angina pectoris, stroke, and total mortality. Death from any cause was also significantly correlated with the ratio of subscapular-to-triceps skinfold (p = 0.046), although the waist-to-hip ratio was a more consistent predictor (p = 0.006). When the women were categorized by quintiles of the waist-to-hip ratio, the risk ratio between the highest quintile and the lowest quintile was 8.2 for myocardial infarction, 3.8 for stroke, and 2.0 for death from any cause. These risk ratios increased to 14.8, 11.0, and 4.8 for the three end points, respectively, when women in the top 5% of the distribution were compared to women in the lowest quintile. For myocardial infarction, angina pectoris, stroke, and total mortality, the waist-to-hip ratio remained a significant risk factor when age, body mass index, and systolic blood pressure were accounted for.

Similar findings were reported for men in Gothenburg who were followed for 13 years [15]. Again, the waist-to-hip ratio was found to be statistically associated with the incidence of stroke, ischemic heart disease, and death from all causes. In contrast to the women, however, a relationship between body mass index or sum of skinfold thicknesses to the three end points was not found. As with the women, the waist-to-hip ratio was found to be related to the incidence of stroke, ischemic heart disease, and death from all causes when the possible confounding effect of body mass index was taken into account. When smoking, systolic blood pressure, and serum cholesterol were considered, however, the ratio was not an independent predictor of the three end points.

In the Paris Prospective Study, a large (n = 6,718) population of men was followed for 6.6 years, and the relationship between fat distribution and the incidence of coronary heart disease was examined [19]. Two independent factors were found to predict coronary heart disease in this population. The first one was a general index of adiposity and the second one opposed skinfolds on the trunk to those on the thigh. The combination of these two factors, interpreted as representing preferential fat deposit on the trunk, mainly on the abdomen, was the best predictor of coronary heart disease risk. The risk was 2.4 times as great for men in the highest quintile of this index compared to those in the lowest quintile. The investigators concluded that trunk-fat deposit, measured by skinfold thicknesses, is a significant predictor of coronary heart disease.

The Framingham Heart Study has reported the contributions of various indices of obesity to the 22-year incidence of coronary heart disease [25]. For men, subscapular skinfold, abdominal skinfold, waist circumference, and body-mass index were all significantly and independently related to the risk of coronary heart disease. The subscapular skinfold measurement was the strongest predictor, while the waist circumference was the weakest. In fact, except for cholesterol, the subscapular skinfold measurement was more highly predictive than any of the other conventional cardiovascular risk factors, including age and systolic blood pressure. For women, only subscapular skinfold and body-mass index served as independent risk factors. The contribution of the waist circumference to coronary heart disease risk declined with age for both sexes. In contrast, the influence of the triceps, abdominal, and thigh skinfolds on risk increased with age for men while the importance of the subscapular skinfold remained fairly consistent by age for women. Most measurements were more predictive for men than they were for women. The hip circumference was not measured in this study, so the relative contribution of the waist-to-hip ratio to coronary heart disease risk could not be determined.

THE INDEPENDENT CONTRIBUTION OF BODY FAT DISTRIBUTION TO BLOOD-PRESSURE LEVEL

Studies on the relationship of body fat distribution to blood pressure have all been cross-sectional, as noted above. These studies have all shown a positive association between upper- or central-body fat distribution and blood pressure. The contribution of body fat distribution to blood pressure was found to be, additionally, independent of total body fat for both men and women in all these studies. Whether the measure of body fat distribution was skinfold thickness measures, skinfold thickness ratios, a waist-to-hip ratio, or other circumference ratios, the data support the existence of a relationship between body-fat distribution and blood pressure independent of fatness itself. Among various measures of body fat distribution, Blair et al. [17] found that although both subscapular and triceps skinfold shared an association with blood pressure, subscapular skinfold had additional predictive power unshared by triceps skinfold. Furthermore, Weinsier et al. [3] found that the subscapular-to-triceps ratio did not significantly increase the power to predict blood-pressure level over the arm-to-thigh ratio.

Prospective studies, including the role of body fat distribution among cardiovascular risk factors, have yielded inconsistent results on the independent effect of fat distribution. The Gothenburg study of women found that the waist-to-hip ratio was a significant risk factor for cardiovascular disease when age, body mass index, and systolic blood pressure were accounted for [14]. Among men in Gothenburg, however, the waist-to-hip ratio was not an independent predictor when smoking, systolic blood pressure, and serum cholesterol were considered, yet was independent of obesity indices [15]. The Paris Prospective Study, on the other hand, found an index combining general adiposity and differential fat deposit to be independently associated with cardiovascular risk, when systolic blood pressure, cholesterol, triglycerides, treatment of diabetes, and smoking were taken into account [19]. Finally, the Framingham Heart Study found various indices of obesity to be significantly and independently related to coronary heart disease risk [25]. Subscapular skinfold was more highly predictive than any of the other obesity indices, although abdominal skinfold, waist circumference, and body mass index also contributed to coronary heart disease risk in men independent of the effect of age, cholesterol, cigarette smoking, systolic blood pressure, blood glucose, and electrocardiographic evidence of left ventricular hypertrophy.

RELATIONSHIP OF BODY FAT DISTRIBUTION TO BLOOD-PRESSURE LEVEL IN NONWHITE POPULATIONS

Comparative data on the relationship between body fat distribution and blood-pressure level in different ethnic groups are valuable in ascribing the relative contributions of diet and genes to central- or upper-body obesity and hypertension. Unfortunately, there are relatively few comparable cross-sectional and prospective studies on body fat distribution and hypertension in nonwhite populations. Blair et al. found that blood pressure level was positively associated with centrally deposited body fat for blacks as well as whites [17]. In a cross-sectional study of American Samoans, the ratio of subscapular skinfold to the sum of triceps and subscapular skinfolds was positively related to both systolic and diastolic blood pressure only among the leanest males [26]. Although there are no prospective studies examining the relationship between body fat distribution and blood pressure level, a recent report from the Honolulu Heart Program indicated that subscapular skinfold thickness was significantly related to the 12-year risk of coronary heart disease among Japanese men independent of overall body fat [27]. These studies seem to validate the relationship between body fat distribution and blood pressure level independent of the influence of ethnicity. This does not by any means negate the fact that some ethnic groups may be more predisposed than others to distribute fat centrally or on the upper body rather than peripherally or on the lower body.

SUMMARY AND CONCLUSIONS

In summary, findings from cross-sectional studies all demonstrate an association between the distribution of body fat and blood pressure. Moreover, a central- or upper-body fat distribution was related to either higher blood-pressure levels or a greater prevalence of hypertension. These studies included large numbers of subjects and a variety of body fat distribution measurements. A number of these studies [3,8,24] dealt with blood pressure as a dichotomous variable (high or normal), while others examined blood pressure as a continuous measure [7,9,17]. In all these studies, the pattern of fat distribution contributed to levels of blood pressure independent of indices of obesity such as body mass index, relative weight, or percentage of body fat.

To determine whether fat patterning is a cause or effect of hypertension, prospective studies are necessary. Unfortunately, there have been no studies to date among adults examining this relationship. Prospective studies of cardiovascular disease have been limited to reports on myocardial infarction, angina pectoris, and stroke. While these studies cannot address the issue of a causal relationship with hypertension, an association between body fat distribution and coronary heart disease may be partly explained by the influence of hypertension as a cardiovascular risk factor. The Gothenburg study demonstrated that, for men, the waist-to-hip ratio was a risk factor for stroke and coronary heart disease, but this relationship was not independent of systolic blood pressure [15]. The Paris Prospective Study, by contrast, found an index interpreted as trunk adiposity to be positively associated with coronary heart disease risk in men, independent of systolic blood pressure [19]. Finally, for women in Gothenburg, the waist-to-hip ratio predicted myocardial infarction, angina pectoris, and stroke, even after taking systolic blood pressure into account [14]. These studies suggest that abdominal obesity carries an increased risk of cardiovascular disease. It is unclear, however, if this risk if totally independent of systolic blood pressure or all other conventional cardiovascular risk factors.

Both upper- and central-body fat predominance have been associated with abdominal obesity. In fact, one study [9] has demonstrated that the waist-to-hip ratio's association with hypertension was mainly due to the influence of the waist circumference, reflecting abdominal fat. Kissebah et al. [6] have shown that upper-body obese individuals have hypertrophy of adipocytes in the abdominal region, while lower-body obese subjects showed smaller abdominal fat cells. These investigators showed that these larger fat cells exhibited a higher rate of lipolysis than fat cells of individuals with lower-body obesity. They suggested that these hypertrophied subcutaneous fat cells may be important due to their high output of free fatty acids to the development of glucose intolerance, hypertriglyceridemia, and hyperinsulinemia among upper-body obese individuals.

Björntorp [28] has hypothesized two routes linking hypertension to abdominal obesity via hyperinsulinemia. One may be due to the action of insulin on increasing renal reabsorption of sodium; the other results from the influence of insulin and carbohydrate metabolism on the sympathetic nervous system activity.

Ashwell [22] has demonstrated, using computed tomography, that the amount of intra-abdominal fat and the ratio of intra-abdominal-to-subcutaneous fat correlates significantly with the waist-to-hip ratio but not with the amount of subcutaneous fat. Thus, the metabolic complications of obesity, which are associated with a high waist-to-hip ratio, may relate more to an excess of intraabdominal fat than to an excess of subcutaneous abdominal fat. This would lend evidence to support the hypothesis of the Gothenburg group who suggest that the relationship of the waist-to-hip ratio to metabolic aberrations may depend on the increased accumulation of intra-abdominal fat cells and their unique position to the portal circulation [7]. The liver is directly exposed to the lipolytic products of the adipocytes in the abdominal depots. Exposure of the liver to excessive levels of free fatty acids has been known to cause hypertriglyceridemia [29]. However, the mechanism by which abdominal obesity may cause hypertension remains unclear.

Since abdominal obesity has been linked to hypertension in cross-sectional studies, cardiovascular disease in prospective studies, and is associated with other established cardiovascular disease risk factors such as diabetes, hypertriglyceridemia, and hyperinsulinemia, the presence of this form of fat patterning should be included as a screening measure for all individuals. Suggested limits for follow-up are a waist-to-hip ratio greater than 1.0 in men and greater than 0.8 in women [28]. Additionally, further studies are needed on the role of body fat distribution in the development of hypertension as well as on the mechanism explaining the hazards of abdominal obesity.

REFERENCES

1. Stamler R, Stamler J, Riedlinger WF, Algera G, Roberts RJ (1978): Weight and blood pressure: findings in hypertension screening of one million Americans. JAMA 240: 1607–1610.
2. Kannel WB, Brand N, Skinner JJ Jr, Dawber TR, McNamara PM (1967): The relation of adiposity to blood pressure and development of hypertension. Ann Intern Med 67: 48–59.
3. Weinsier RL, Norris DJ, Birch R, Bernstein RS, Wang J, Yang M-U, Pierson, Jr. RN, Van Itallie TB (1985): The relative contribution of body fat and fat pattern to blood pressure level. Hypertension 7:578–585.

4. Weinsier RL, Fuchs RJ, Kay TD, Triebwasser JH, Lancaster MC (1976): Body fat: its relationship to coronary heart disease, blood pressure, lipids and other risk factors measured in a large male population. Am J Med 61:815–824.

5. Robinson SC, Brucer M (1940): Body build and hypertension. Arch Intern Med 66: 393–417.

6. Kissebah AH, Vydelingum N, Murray R, Evans D, Hartz AJ, Kalkhoff RK, Adams PW (1982): Relationship of body fat distribution to metabolic complications of obesity. J Clin Endocrinol Metab 54:254–260.

7. Krotkiewski M, Björntorp P, Sjöström L, Smith U (1983): Impact of obesity on metabolism in men and women: importance of regional adipose tissue distribution. J Clin Invest 72:1150–1162.

8. Hartz AJ, Rupley DC, Rimm AA (1984): The association of girth measurements with disease in 32,856 women. Am J Epidemiol 119:71–80.

9. Kalkhoff RK, Hartz AJ, Rupley D, Kissebah AH, Kelber S (1983): Relationship of body fat distribution to blood pressure, carbohydrate tolerance, and plasma lipids in healthy obese women. J Lab Clin Med 102:621–627.

10. Vague J (1956): The degree of masculine differentiation of obesities: a factor determining predisposition to diabetes, atherosclerosis, gout, and uric calculous disease. Am J Clin Nutr 4:20–34.

11. Stern MP, Haffner SM (1986): Body fat distribution and hyperinsulinemia as risk factors for diabetes and cardiovascular disease. Arteriosclerosis 6:123–130.

12. Feldman R, Sender AJ, Siegelaub AB (1969): Difference in diabetic and nondiabetic fat distribution patterns by skinfold measurements. Diabetes 18:478–486.

13. Szathmary EJE, Holt N (1983): Hyperglycemia in Dogrib Indians of the Northwest Territories, Canada: association with age and a centripetal distribution of body fat. Hum Biol 55:493–515.

14. Lapidus L, Bengtsson C, Larsson B, Pennert K, Rybo E, Sjöström L (1984): Distribution of adipose tissue and risk of cardiovascular disease and death: a 12 year follow up of participants in the population study of women in Gothenburg, Sweden. Br Med J 289: 1257–1261.

15. Larsson B, Svärdsudd K, Welin L (1984): Abdominal adipose tissue distribution, obesity, and risk of cardiovascular disease and death: 13 year follow up of participants in the study of men born in 1913. Br Med J 288:1401–1404.

16. Gerber LM, Madhavan S, Alderman MH (1987): Waist-to-hip ratio as an index of risk for hyperglycemia among hypertensive patients. Am J Prev Med 3:64–68.

17. Blair D, Habicht JP, Sims EAH, Sylwester D, Abraham S (1984): Evidence for an increased risk for hypertension with centrally located body fat and the effect of race and sex on this risk. Am J Epidemiol 119:526–540.

18. Mueller WH, Wohlleb JC (1981): Anatomical distribution of subcutaneous fat and its description by multivariate methods: How valid are the principal components? Am J Phys Anthr 54:25–35.

19. Ducimetiere P, Richard J, Cambien F (1986): The pattern of subcutaneous fat distribution in middle-aged men and the risk of coronary heart disease: The Paris Prospective Study. Int J Obesity 10:229–240.

20. Hartz AJ, Rupley DC, Kalkhoff RD, Rimm AA (1983): Relationship of obesity to diabetes: influence of obesity level and body fat distribution. Prev Med 12:351–357.

21. Shuman WP, Newell Morris LL, Leonetti DL, Wahl PW, Moceri VM, Moss AA, Fujimoto WY (1986): Abdominal body fat distribution detected by computed tomography in diabetic men. Invest Radiol 21:483–487.

22. Ashwell M, Cole TJ, Dixon AK (1985): Obesity: new insight into the anthropometric

classification of fat distribution shown by computed tomography. Br Med J 290:1692–1694.

22. Borkan GA, Gerzof SG, Robbins AH, Hults DE, Silbert CK, Silbert JE (1982): Assessment of abdominal fat content by computed tomography. Am J Clin Nutr 36:172–177.

23. Seidell JC, Bakx JC, DeBoer E, Deurenberg P, Hautvast JGAJ (1985): Fat distribution of overweight persons in relation to morbidity and subjective health. Int J Obes 9: 363–374.

24. Stokes J III, Garrison RJ, Kannel WB (1985): The independent contributions of various indices of obesity to the 22-year incidence of coronary heart disease: The Framingham Heart Study. In Vague J, et al. (eds): "Metabolic Complications of Human Obesities." New York: Elsevier, pp 49–57.

25. McGarvey ST (1984): Subcutaneous fat distribution and blood pressure of Samoans. Paper presented at the 1984 meeting of the American Association of Physical Anthropologists, Philadelphia, Pennsylvania, April 12–14.

26. Donahue RP, Abbott RD, Bloom E, Reed DM, Yano K (1987): Central obesity and coronary heart disease in men. Lancet i:821–824.

27. Björntorp P (1985): Obesity and the risk of cardiovascular disease. Ann Clin Res 17:3–9.

28. Carlsson LA, Boberg J, Högstedt B. (1965): Some physiological and clinical implications of lipid mobilization from adipose tissue. Handb Physiol 5:625–644.

Nutritional Factors in Hypertension
© 1990 Alan R. Liss, Inc., pages 79–95

6 | Nutritional Approaches to Hypertension

J. Wylie-Rosett Ed.D., R.D.
C. Swencionis, Ph.D.

INTRODUCTION

There are a wide range of choices available to control blood pressure [1–4]. Over 60 medications and a wide variety of dietary approaches can be used [1–3]. There appears to be a consensus that moderate elevation of blood pressure should be treated and that even mild hypertension should be carefully treated with nonpharmacological therapy [2]. The 1984 Joint National Committee on Detection, Evaluation and Treatment of High Blood Pressure recommended that if an individual has a diastolic blood pressure over 90 mmHg or a systolic measurement over 160 mmHg that there should be repeated blood pressure measurements and, if the pressure remains elevated, treatment is needed [1]. These guidelines have been updated in 1988 to include information from recent hypertension clinical trials [3]. However, selecting the most appropriate therapy for a patient with hypertension still remains difficult for the clinician. Most people with elevated blood pressure are being treated. However, it appears that achieving adequate blood pressure control is more difficult in the usual practice of medicine, as noted in the evaluation of usual community care results the Hypertension Detection and Follow-Up Program [5], and more recently in the impact of antihypertensive therapy on lipids and cardiovascular risk has been questioned based on the Multiple Risk Factor Intervention Trial [6].

From the Department of Epidemiology/Social Medicine, Albert Einstein College of Medicine, and Ferknauf Graduate School of Psychology of Yeshiva University, Bronx, NY 10461.

Dietary intervention was the only treatment available until the 1950s, when the thiazide diuretics and other pharmacologic agents were introduced. With the advent of drug therapy, there was less emphasis on dietary approaches. The decreased use of dietary approaches may have been partially related to the severity of early dietary restrictions such as the Kempner diet, which consists solely of boiled rice and fruit. Concern about the side effects of medications and their impact on quality of life has renewed interest in dietary treatment of blood pressure. Each of the nutrient variables is covered as the theme of other chapters in this book. Chapters deal with sodium, potassium, and obesity respectively.

This chapter will provide an overview of the dietary methods focusing on the translation of epidemiological and physiological research into clinical trials that demonstrate efficacy. Criteria for selecting a dietary approach in various clinical environments will be discussed, as will be approaches to changing dietary habits. All antihypertensive regimens require behavioral changes, and approaches to behavioral change will be discussed.

OVERVIEW OF DIETARY APPROACHES

There appears to be general agreement that nutritional habits are related to the prevalence of hypertension and that dietary modification can be used to treat hypertension [2]. However, which dietary variables affect blood pressure and the best dietary treatment approach is a source of considerable debate. Sodium restriction and weight control are closely linked epidemiologically to hypertension and are widely used treatment approaches [2,6–30]. Several nutrients have become of interest more recently based on epidemiological evidence that associates a higher intake with a lower rate of hypertension or clinical studies using dietary modification or supplements. These nutrients include potassium [2,6,27–29], magnesium [2,32,34], calcium [2,30–34], linoleic acid [34], omega-3 fatty acids [35], and fiber [36]. The statistical and possible physiological interaction of nutrients has completed identification of a single approach to nutrient therapy in hypertension [37]. Excessive intake of alcohol [2,11–13,19,20,26,33] is associated with a rise in blood pressure and with hypertriglyceridemia, and cessation or reduction in its use has been used to help control hypertension. Combinations of these approaches are also being used in clinical trials that are studying hypertension prevention or treatment. Table 1 lists each approach prevalence or of action, customary intake, typical intervention dietary modification and problems in achieving or evaluating the dietary modification.

Sodium

The sodium intake of a society is related to the prevalence rate of hypertension [1–3,7–11]. However, whether excess sodium intake is a direct cause

Table 1. Nutritional Therapy of Hypertension

Established approaches	Intake prevalence in U.S.	Level used to treat BP	Issues related to Success of Intervention
Sodium restriction	7 to 15 gm is the usual sodium intake for Americans	< 2gm	Omitting of convience foods and condiments will reduce intake to a 300 mg. achieving a intake of <2000 mg is difficult. Treatment may be effective for mild hypertensive patients but not for others.
Weight control	40 million Americans are considered to be overweight.	Loss of 10–15 lbs. may control BP	Treatment is appealing and may help with other risk factors. Appears to be best dietary approach for overweight hypertensive patients.
Alcohol restrictions	Moderate intake is estimated to be less than 2 ounces ETOH per day.	< 2 ounces of ethyl alcohol	Is likely to be highly effective in those consuming high levels. Obtaining intake information may be difficult.
Experimental approaches			
Potassium (dietary increase or supplements)	40–50 mEq	> 80 mEq	Achieving dietary intake above 60 mEq is difficult. Supplements may cause gastrointestinal problems.
Calcium (dietary) increase or supplements	400–600 mg	> 1 gram	Increasing dietary intake may be difficult High intake may increase risk calcium based renal stones in susceptible individuals.
Fat modification	Typical fatty acid intake: polyunsaturated 4 to 5% of total calories Monosaturated Saturated	Prudent diet monosaturated omega-3 fatty acids dose is about 4% of calories in	Diet may have other benefits, i.e., reduction in cholesterol or platelet aggregation. Use of omega-3 supplement may pose other risk, i.e., environmental toxins, prolonged bleeding in patients on an anticoagulant.
Magnesium			Increasing dietary intake may be difficult. There is insufficient evidence to justify the use of supplements
Fiber dietary	7 gm/1000 calories	Not established for BP 25 gm/1000 calories up to 40–50 grams as recommended in diabetes.	Increasing dietary intake may be difficult. Supplements may cause gastrointestinal distress.

of hypertension or sodium restriction is the most effective approach to dietary modification to control high blood pressure is less clear [2,14–17]. The level of sodium restriction that is required to effectively reduce blood pressure has been evaluated. Prior to the introduction of drug therapy, the goal for sodium restriction was usually less than 500 mg per day, and many of the patients had malignant hypertension that was poorly controlled. The impact of moderate sodium restriction on blood pressure is somewhat controversial. The average intake of sodium in the United States is thought to be between 5 and 15 gm. A moderate sodium restriction is approximately 2000 mg; a limit of 3000 milligrams has been recommended by the American Heart Association for the general public [19]. Processed foods are the primary source of dietary sodium, with bread and grain products such as cereal being the largest contributor to sodium intake. Reducing sodium intake to approximately 2500 to 3000 milligrams may be achieved by elimination of discretionary sodium sources such as added salt and fast foods, and reeducation in use of convenience foods and condiments. Achieving an intake goal of less than 2500 milligrams may be difficult in general clinical practice. However, in clinical trials participants report an intake of 1500 to 2000 mg with mean urinary excretion that is about 20% higher than self-reported dietary estimates, possibly indicating that patients "think" they are more successful than the objective laboratory measures [16,38].

Obesity and Weight Control

Obesity is closely linked to elevation of blood pressure. Weight control is becoming of increasing importance in the study and possible treatment of hypertension [2,12–23]. There is growing evidence of multiple benefits for weight control in overweight hypertensive patients [2,24,38]. Reducing body weight appears to reduce insulin resistance and lower blood pressure. The mechanism by which weight reduction lowers blood pressure appears to involve hormonal regulation [24]. Although calorie restriction has been demonstrated to reduce blood pressure, it is often associated with a concomitant decrease in the intake of sodium. As a result, there was some question as to whether weight control in itself lowered blood pressure. It has been demonstrated that even when the sodium level is kept constant, weight reduction lowers blood pressure [25]. Indeed, in obese individuals weight control appears to be more effective in maintaining blood pressure in individuals with moderate hypertension after they have been tapered off antihypertensive medication [16,21]. The reduction in blood pressure and/or the ability to be maintained free of antihypertensive medication appears to be maintained after the weight stabilizes. Weight control may also help reduce cardiovascular risk in several ways that are independent of its effect on blood pressure. A higher high-density lipoprotein (HDL) and possibly a lower total and low-density lipoprotein (LDL) cholesterol may be associated with weight reduction, as is a lower blood glucose in diabetic individuals. However, whether these cholesterol changes are maintained long term needs further study.

Weight control may also appeal to the patient with hypertension for cosmetic and personal reasons. Preliminary results from Trial of Antihypertensive Intervention and Management (TAIM) indicate that weight-control participants judge that their quality of life improves following weight-reduction intervention. This may be in part due to the behavioral appraoch used that evaluates quality of life in detail.

Potassium

There has been interest in the possible role of potassium in the prevention and treatment of hypertension. Potassium supplementation is frequently used with thiazide diuretic therapy. The role of potassium in controlling blood pressure is not fully determined, but there are some studies that have shown a small but significant fall in blood pressure as the result of potassium supplementation [27–29]. Many of the supplements are associated with gastrointestinal distress [2]. However, attempts to raise potassium by diet may result in only a modest increase in intake. Traditionally, orange juice and bananas were the foods that patients were told to eat to increase dietary potassium. Foods such as legumes, whole grains, potatoes, tomatoes, and broccoli also can be used to increase dietary potassium.

Calcium

The relationship between calcium intake and blood pressure is of considerable interest [31–34]. Several studies have shown an inverse relationship between calcium intake and blood pressure, and calcium supplementation has been shown to reduce blood pressure. However, more research is needed to understand the effect on blood pressure. Attempts to increase dietary calcium may not have resulted in a substantial increase in calcium intake. Dairy products are the primary source of dietary calcium, and data from the National Health and Nutrition Examination Survey suggest that most Americans are below the recommended intake for this nutrient [12,13]. Indeed, much of the original interest in calcium with respect to blood pressure has related to analysis of NHANES data.

More recently, magnesium has become of interest with respect to the eliology and possible treatment of elevated blood pressure [2,32,34]. Increasing dietary magnesium may be difficult. The best food sources of magnesium are nuts and whole grains, followed in value by vegetables and fruits. When intake of these foods is increased, dietary potassium is also increased.

More research is needed to evaluate the impact of magnesium supplementation and to assess potential mechanisms of action.

Fat and Fatty Acids

Diets that are low in fat and/or those with a high polyunsaturated-to-saturated fat ratio have been shown to reduce blood pressure in a population [2,34,35]. Polyunsaturated fatty acids appear to alter prostaglandin synthesis and may be the primary cause of the blood pressure lowering effect of a prudent diet. However, many individuals also reduce sodium intake and calories as part of a prudent dietary intake, and these changes are also likely to reduce blood pressure. More recently, there has been interest in the blood pressure lowering potential of the omega-3 fatty acids [35]. Since these fatty acids are polyunsaturated, the potential mechanism of action for lowering blood pressure is likely to be related to prostaglandin synthesis.

Fiber

Dietary fiber has also been suggested to possibly lower blood pressure as well as blood glucose [36]. Whether dietary fiber has a direct effect on blood pressure remains to be determined. If fiber reduces insulin resistance in conjunction with its blood glucose lowering effect, it may also reduce blood pressure through a similar mechanism to that proposed for weight reduction. Food sources of dietary fiber are freqeuently high in potassium, which may also have a blood pressure lowering effect.

Alcohol

A high alcohol intake has been associated with hypertension, and reduction in intake appears to lower blood pressure [2,13]. The American Heart Association [19] and the Subcommittee on Nonpharmacological Approaches of the Joint National Committee [2] recommend limiting daily alcohol intake to less than two ounces of alcohol. Although excess alcohol intake may be involved in the etiology of the hypertension for a small subset of those with elevated blood pressure, cessation of alcohol is clearly the first-line treatment for anyone who is a heavy drinker and has hypertension. Intake level for some individuals may be provided more readily on a nutritional history than on direct questioning about potential alcohol abuse. For the obese individual who consumes more than two ounces of ethanol per day, elimination of or reduction in alcohol intake may reduce body weight [2,19,24]. Reduction in alcohol intake may also result in weight loss.

SELECTING AN INTERVENTION APPROACH

The controversy over the roles of various nutrients in the development treatment of high blood pressure indicates the need for further research and clinical trials to determine the "best treatment" for hypertension. However, there is strong evidence to support intervention to control hypertension, and there is growing evidence that clinicians need to consider dietary intervention as an adjunct or as an alternative to the pharmacological treatment of elevated blood pressure. Concerns over the side effects of medication and quality-of-life issues have renewed interest in dietary treatment. These research debates should not deter the use of dietary approaches, and the selection of a dietary approach needs to consider the physiological factors such as weight and other cardiovascular risk factors, the health care setting, nutritional history, and behavioral issues.

Physiological Factors

The treatment approach to hypertension is largely determined by the severity of the blood pressure elevation. Dietary intervention alone may be enough to control mild hypertension but is unlikely to control greater degrees of blood pressure elevation. There may be a wide range of responsiveness to dietary modification. However, the amount of antihypertensive medication needed may be reduced if dietary intervention is used concomitantly, thus reducing the drug side effects. Some individuals may not physiologically respond to dietary modification, making them "hyporespond," while the blood pressure of others may be quite responsive to dietary change, making them "hyperresponders."

Obese individuals may be more amenable to a dietary approach that emphasizes weight reduction. The cosmetic effects may make this approach quite acceptable. When there are other weight-related cardiovascular risk factors such as diabetes, the emphasis on weight reduction becomes more critical, and weight loss may also raise HDL cholesterol and reduce triglycerides. For the lean individual with elevated blood pressure, reduction in sodium may be effective. However, if there are other health problems that would benefit for the less-well-established approaches, their potential effect on blood pressure should be considered. However, because the impacts of some of these dietary modifications require further investigation, their use should focus on potential secondary benefits.

If blood cholesterol is elevated, the emphasis may be more appropriately placed on modification of fat intake. For the lean individual with diabetes, emphasis on dietary fiber may be warranted. When the medication intervention includes diuretics, evaluation of potassium is needed and should focus on a wide range of foods and not be limited to orange juice and bananas. Obviously, for individuals with excessive alcohol intake, the focus needs to include the potential benefit on blood pressure or reducing or eliminating alcohol intake. For the woman who has been identified at risk for osteoporosis and who has an inadequate calcium intake, it may be reasonable to consider the potential blood pressuring lowering effect of calcium.

Nutrition History

The probability of achieving success with a dietary approach in hypertension may be determined by the present intake and willingness and/or ability to modify intake. For the lean individual who follows a prudent diet with a sodium intake of less than 100 mEq, there is less likelihood of physiological response to dietary modification than for the individual who has more dietary excess. However, the individual who has a greater potential for a physiological response may be less likely to make dietary changes.

Previous experience with dietary modification can help guide the selection of a dietary approach. If a similar dietary approach has been used previously, the degree of dietary modification and responsiveness may be important in assessing whether using the same approach is likely to be effective. In the treatment of obesity, an individual and family weight history is needed to help determine the milieu in which the weight program will be introduced. Family and individual attitudes and beliefs about weight and weight control are also important.

Achieving Dietary Change

Motivation and stages of dietary change may be important for understanding the psychological processes involved. Prochaska and DiClemente [39] divided smoking cessation into stages with verbal and behavioral processes within them. Dietary change is quite different from smoking cessation, but both have addictive components, and it is likely that similar motivational components apply. They propose five stages: 1) contemplation, 2) deciding to change, 3) action, 4) maintenance, and 5) relapse. The relapse may lead back to an earlier stage, leading to further attempts at change, in a circular rather than a linear model.

One use of such a model might be to assess an individual's readiness for change, screening out those not currently ''ripe'' and making suggestions as to how individuals could work on their own motivation and return at a more propitious time. This has serious ethical implications. It is highly desirable to screen out those who will fail at nutritional change, but unethical to screen out those who the screening indicates will fail but who would in fact succeed.

APPROACHES TO COUNSELING

Problem Identification

A behavioral approach to counseling is oriented around identifying specific goals and then working toward them. Seldom does the patient state problems in a clear and specific enough manner to allow work immediately. The first responsibility of the behavioral counselor is to help the client identify the problems [40]. The counselor does this by listening closely to what the client is saying to understand and be able to analyze specific parts of the behaviors the client is involved in. For example, does the problem begin with making up the grocery list, in the grocery store, food preparation with particular food groups at certain times, or places and circumstances of eating? Listening, trying to clarify perceptions of what the patient is experiencing, and trying to reconstruct the behavior sequence that leads to problems will reveal weak links in chains of behavior where intervention can be helpful.

Goal Setting

The client always sets his or her own goals, with the counselor only advising. Setting large goals, such as the loss of a certain amount of weight per week, can be easy, with the counselor advising as to what is possible.

PSYCHOLOGICAL FACTORS

Psychological assessment to determine the best antihypertensive nutritional approach for an individual or group is not very advanced. As in other areas of health psychology, psychological methods have been developed to address problems of psychopathology and retardation, while a different range of function must be addressed here. These are psychologically "normal" people who have problems with eating and physical activity behaviors.

Few formal or specific assessment procedures have been developed for these nutritional interventions. However, there is considerable psychological experience with weight-reduction treatments and some with sodium restriction and potassium elevation.

WEIGHT REDUCTION

Behavioral treatment of obesity leads to consistent weight loss of 10 to 11 pounds which is maintained at 1 year [41–43]. While such losses may be of limited value to the morbidly obese, they do produce decreases in blood pressure in most hypertensive people over ideal weight. Wadden [44] has noticed no additional blood pressure drop beyond 15 lbs. loss.

Techniques of behavioral treatment of obesity are described in several reviews [42,45–49]. Wilson and Brownell [44] reviewed 17 long-term studies and found a mean attrition rate of 13.5%. In studies that used a deposit-refund system, attrition was 9.5%, and in other studies it averaged 19.3%.

MOTIVATION

Long a dormant area of psychology, motivation is returning to vogue as change among health-related behaviors is studied more and more. What can be more difficult is subgoals, such as identifying that it is snacks before bedtime which are the problem. The following are some commonly encountered problems in dealing with subgoals.

"The Problem Is Someone Else's Behavior"

For example, "My husband keeps ice cream in the freezer and I can't resist it." In this situation, the nutritionist counselor must identify the client as the person being seen, not the spouse, unless the client has brought the spouse in. Additionally, the client can be helped to see what kinds of behavior to engage in to remedy the difficulty. The client's behavior can be worked with directly, but the client can learn that others' behavior can be changed by the same principles.

The Problem Expressed As a Feeling

For example, "I eat when I feel lonely." Two strategies for dealing with this are: (a) engaging in behavior incompatible with the undesired feeling; and (b) changing standards for comparing feelings. To engage in incompatible behaviors might require a social skills training course, or counseling beyond what a nutritionist might be capable of. A psychologist providing supervision might be extremely helpful. Overbroad problems, such as "I eat when I feel depressed," are not an answer, and require further discussion to become more precise. Establishing more realistic standards is facilitated in a group, where members find others share their feelings. However, any unrealistic standards, such as expecting cosmetic appearance secondary to weight loss to be improved enormously after a week or two, must be pointed out by any counselor as unrealistic and resulting in disappointment.

The Desired Behavior Is Undesirable

The client may have an excessively rigid, extreme notion of how to reach a goal—for example, to eat only fruit to raise potassium and decrease sodium. This is similar to setting unrealistic goals in that the counselor must advise what is unrealistic.

Revision of goals. Goals should continually be reviewed. Progress is assessed in terms of meeting or advancing toward goals, but goals can be changed. If a client sets a 2 lb/week weight-loss goal and fails to meet it two weeks in succession, it is time to renegotiate the goal downward to reflect a more realistic goal. Otherwise, the client will always feel frustrated and lose interest. This is true of behavioral as well as physiological goals. If a client feels "burned out" from excessive striving after good progress, one might suggest a week's vacation from further gains, being careful to maintain present levels without backsliding.

Support. Many studies have shown the positive effects of social support on nutritional and on other kinds of behavior change. The more the spouse or other family members can be brought in to the intervention, even coming to sessions, the better.

Cognitive strategies. In addition to behavioral change, cognitive change is important. The phrases that people say to themselves mentally have effects on what they do. For example, "I can't lose weight," "I can't change what I eat." Such repetitive phrases should be noted as they come up in counseling. Their existence, their irrationality, and the effects they have can be pointed out, and substitute ones can be suggested, such as "I have already lost _____pounds," or "I have already learned to eat more fruit."

BARRIERS TO ADHERENCE

The topics listed in Table 2 emerge repeatedly in nutritional counseling. We do not suggest simple solutions, but only that these topics require clinical and research attention. Better solutions to these problems will produce more effective nutritional counseling interventions, and maintenance of change. This list was generated from interviews with patients in clinical trials who had been on weight reduction, sodium restriction, and potassium elevation regimens. Some interviews were conducted after the trial—the Hypertension Prevention Trial (HPT)—was completed, and others were results of content analyses performed on nutritionists' notes of individual sessions during a trial (TAIM).

MAINTENANCE AND RELAPSE

Maintenance of changes and prevention and treatment of relapse have become a defined area of research and treatment of addictive behaviors. Food may be different from smoking and drug use in that one should not cease eating, but it has strong addictive components. Marlatt and Gordon [50] presented a theoretical schema for understanding and dealing with relapse. Brownell et al. [51] review this and other formulations of relapse and maintenance. Although this is a new and active area of research, some statements can be made.

Extended Contact

Some provision for extended contact should be present. The Multiple risk Factor Intervention Trial [52], which had an excellent record of maintenance

Table 2. Barriers to Adherence Noted in Nutrition Counseling

A. *Motivation*
  1. The client expects someone else to treat them, that they
     can be passive, and that the interventionist will do all
     the work.
  2. Lack of follow-through
B. *Social Stressors*
  1. Excessive job demands on time
  2. Other demands on time
  3. Travel
  4. Frequent eating out
C. *Interpersonal*
  1. Spousal resistance
  2. Lack of support from significant others
  3. Cooking for others
D. *Self-Regulatory and Emotional*
  1. Unrealistic goals
  2. Not self-monitoring
  3. Uses food to reward or comfort self, eats when upset,
     bored, or stressed
  4. Does not structure intervention into lifestyle
  5. Evening snacking
E. *Food Planning, Preparation, and Choice*
  1. Does not prepare foods
  2. Limited variety of foods
  3. Eats mostly convenience (snack or fast) foods
  4. Menu planning
  5. Does not do shopping or shops when hungry, does not
     read labels
  6. Excessive condiment use
  7. Fried foods
F. *Addictive Components of Foods*
  1. Eat too fast or always feels hungry
  2. Tempted by foods, cravings
  3. Eats large portions, or multiple portions.
  4. Alcohol use
G. *Physical Activity*
  1. Perceived disability
  2. Dislikes or fails to schedule physical activity

and low relapse rate, maintained contact at least every 6 weeks with participants, and more frequently with those who had more difficulties following the regimen. Booster sessions, however, which repeat the principles learned earlier, are generally ineffective in smoking cessation [53,54]. Follow-up sessions should be geared to solving current problems, and continued monitoring and vigilance are essential.

Abstinence Violation

Marlatt and Gordon [50] determined that the response to lapse or relapse may be to say, "I've slipped, why not go all out?" Clients may be prepared for lapse or relapse by rehearsal of what to do in the event of a slip, so that they can self-correct. The most extreme form of this, and rather controversial, is programmed lapse, where the client is instructed to lapse and to recover from it in a certain way. The discrimination of lapse from relapse is also important. A lapse can be one or several small slips, which the client learns from, and returns to the regimen. A relapse is more serious, and may lead to giving up entirely.

Addictive Eating and Emotional Problems

Targeting specific problem foods and developing individualized strategies for them may be helpful. It is very helpful to have psychological supervision available so that the nutritional counselor does not get beyond his or her depth. Referral may be necessary.

Physical Activity

As a positive addiction, exercise may have a special role in restructuring eating behaviors, changing set point, and changing body percepts.

Ongoing Problem Solving

Although rehashing of initial intervention techniques has not been helpful, reconsideration of all of them in the context of how they are failing in the present can be helpful. For example, what can be done to change social support, cognitive restructuring, integration of lifestyle change, and other principles used in initial intervention. Key to this approach is analysis of what the problems are at the moment for the client. Careful study of this will lead to a natural history of relapse and maintenance.

HEALTH CARE SETTING

Treatment approach is greatly affected by the health care setting. The availability of nutrition services needs to be evaluated and the evaluation should include a qualitative assessment of the counseling. For example, if a patient will only receive a written list of foods to eat and those to avoid, the impact of dietary intake is likely to be minimal. However, there are a growing number of registered dietitians available for referrals in private practice and in medical groups. For weight reeducation counseling there is a variety of commercial programs that offer follow-up and a well-balanced approach to dietary modification.

If counseling is approached as a two step process, many physicians and nurses could provide some basic nutrition counseling education and a referral to a dietitian could be made for in-depth counseling.

Many people find food less interesting after being told that dietary modification is need to control cardiovascular or health risks. Local American Heart Association affiliates often offer cooking courses and may have a local restaurant guide.

CONCLUSIONS

Nutritional treatment of hypertension is a valuable adjunct to pharmacotherapy and in some cases is adequate by itself. There are many approaches which must be chosen among and tailored to the individual, group, or institutional situation. The best demonstrated approaches are weight reduction, sodium restriction, and potassium elevation. Other approaches are promising but more experimental.

Nutritional approaches are enjoying a resurgence of interest because they can reduce or sometimes even eliminate the need for drug therapy, thus reducing side effects and enhancing quality of life. Quality-of-life issues need to be carefully examined in nutritional regimens as well, because people may find nutritional regimens restrictive.

The wider variety of nutritional approaches now available, and advances in nutritional counseling which have taken place in the last 40 years, make this a promising developing area of treatment.

REFERENCES

1. Joint National Committee on Detection Evaluation and Treatment of High Blood Pressure (1984): The 1984 Report of the Joint National Committee on Detection Evaluation and Treatment of High Blood Pressure. Arch Intern Med 144:1045–1057.
2. Subcommittee on Non-Pharmacological Approaches to the Control of High Blood Pressure of the 1984 Joint National Committee on Detection, Evaluation and Treatment of High Blood Pressure (1986): Non-Pharmacological approaches to the control of high blood pressure. Hypertension 8:444–467.
3. The 1988 Report of the Joint National Committee of Detection, Evaluation and Treatment of High Blood Pressure, Arch Intern Med, Vol. 148, May 1988; 1023–1038.
4. Physicians Desk Reference (PDR) 4158 Editor Oradell, NJ Medical Economics Inc, 43 edition, 1989.
5. Hypertension Detection and Follow-up Program Group (1982): The effect of treatment on mortality in mild hypertension: Results of the hypertension detection and follow-up program. N Engl J Med 307:976–980.
6. Cagiulla AW: A new challenge for antihypertensive therapy: Total cardiovascular risk factor reduction. In: Wasserthiel-Smoller S, Wylie-Rosett J (eds): Cardiovascular Health Risk Assessment and Risk Management 1989.
7. Altschul AM, Grommet JK (1980): Sodium intake and sodium sensitivity. Nutr Rev 38:393–402.

8. Kempner W (1948): Treatment of cardiovascular disease with rice diet. Am J Med 4: 545–547.

9. Dahl LK (1961): Possible note of chronic excess salt consumption in the pathogenesis of essential hypertension. Am J Cardiol 8:571–75.

10. Weinsier RL (1976). Overview: salt and the development of essential hypertension. Prev Med 1976;5:7–14.

11. Freis ED (1976): Salt Volume and the prevention of hypertension. Circulation 53:589–595.

12. Harlan WR, Hull AL, Schmounder RL, Landis R, Thompson FE, Larkin FA (1984): Blood pressure and nutrition in adults: The National Health and Nutrition Examination Survey. Am J Epidemiol 120:17–28.

13. McCarron DA, Morris CD, Henry HJ, Stanton JL (1984): Blood pressure and nutrient intake in the United States. Science 224:1392–1398.

14. Gruchow HW, Sobocinski KA, Barboriak JJ (1985): Alcohol nutrient intake and hypertension in U.S. adults. JAMA 253:1567–1570.

15. Kaplan NM (1985): Non-drug treatment of hypertension. Ann Intern Med 102:359–373.

16. Horan MJ, Blaustein MP, Dunbar JB, Grundy S, Kachadorian W, Kaplan NM, Kotchen TA, Simopoulos AP, Van Italie TB (1985): NIH Report on research challenges in nutrition and hypertension. Hypertension 7:818–23.

17. Wasserthiel-Smoller S, Langford HG, Blaufox MD, Oberman A, Hawkins M, Levine B, Cameron M, Babcock C, Pressel S, Caggiula A, Cutter G, Curb D, Wing R (1985): Effective dietary intervention in hypertension: Sodium restriction and weight reduction. J Am Dietet Assoc 85:423–430.

18. Stamler R, Stanter J, Grimm R, Dyer A, Gosch F, Berman R, Elmer P, Fishman J, Van Heel N, Civinelli J, Hosekema R (1985): Nonpharmacological control of hypertension. Prev Med 14:336–345.

19. American Heart Association: Dietary Guidelines for Healthy American Adults, 1986, circulation.

20. MacGregor GA (1985): Sodium is more important than calcium in essential hypertension. Hypertension 7:628–637.

21. Langford HG, Blaufox MD, Oberman A, Hawkins CM, Curb JD, Cutter GR, Wassertheil-Smoller S, Pressel S, Babcock C, Abernathy SD, Hotchkiss J, Tyler M (1985): Diet therapy slows the return of hypertension after with stopping prolonged medication JAMA 253:657–664.

22. Morgan T, Gilles A, Morgan G, Adam W, Wilson M, Carney S (1978): Hypertension Treated by salt restriction. Lancet February, 1:227–30.

23. Stamler J, Farinaro F, Mojonnier LM, Hall Y, Moss D, Stamler R (1980): Prevention and control of hypertension by nutritional-hygienic means. JAMA 243:1819–1823.

24. Maxwell MH, Waks AW: Obesity and hypertension. In HG Langford, MD Blaufox (eds): Bibl Cardiol No. 41, Karger, New York, 1987. ''Nonpharmacological Therapy of Hypertension'' pp 29–39.

25. Reisen E, Abel R, Modan B, Silverberg DS, Eliahow HE, Modan B (1981): Effect of weight loss without self restriction or the reduction of blood pressure in overweight hypertensive patients. N Engl J Med 298:1–10.

26. Calloway WC (1983): Nutritional factors and blood pressure control: An assessment. Ann Intern Med 98 (part 2):884–890.

27. Langford HG (1987): Potassium and its role in the etiology and therapy of hypertension. Bibl Cardiol No. 41, Karger, New York, 1987. In Langford, HG Blaufox MD (eds): ''Non-pharmacological Therapy of Hypertension.'' Karger, Basel: 41:57–68.

28. MacGregor G (1983): Dietary sodium and potassium intake and blood pressure. Lancet 1:750–53.

29. Treasure J, Ploth D (1983): Role of dietary potassium in the treatment of hypertension. Hypertension 5:864–872.
30. McCarron DA (1987): Is calcium more important than sodium in the pathogenesis of essential hypertension? Hypertension 7:607–627.
31. Belizan JM, Villar J, Pineda O, Gonzalez AE, Sainz E, Garrera G, Sibrian R (1983): Reduction of blood pressure with calcium supplementation in young adults. JAMA 249: 1161–1165.
32. McCarron DA (1983): Calcium and magnesium nutrition and human hypertension. Annals Intern Med 98 (part 2):800–805.
33. Stanton JL, Braitman LE, Riley AM, Khoo CS, Smith JL (1982): Demography dietary life style and anthropometric correlates of blood pressure. Hypertension 4:Supp.III:135–142.
34. Weinsier RL, Norris D (1985): Recent developments in the etiology and treatment of hypertension: Dietary calcium, fat and magnesium. Am J Clin Nutr 42:1331–1338.
35. Herold PM, Kinessa JE: Fish oil consumption and decreased risk of cardiovascular disease: A comparison of finding from animal and human feeding trials. Am J Clin Nutr 43:566.36.
36. Anderson JW (1983): Plant fiber and blood pressure. Ann Intern Med 98:842–846.
37. Reed D, McGee D, Yango K, Hankin J (1983): Diet Blood Pressure and Multicollinearity. Hypertension 7:405–410.
38. Cagiulla AW, Milas NC, Wing RR (1987): Optimal nutritional therapy in the treatment on hypertension. In HG Langford, MD Blaufox (eds): "Non-Pharmacological Therapy of Hypertension." Kargel, Basel: Biblthca Cardiol 41:6–21.
39. Prochaska JO, DiClemente CC (1983): Stages and processes of self-change of smoking: Toward an integrative model of change. Consult Clin Psychol 51:390–395.
40. Krumbolz JD, Thoresen CE (eds.) (1969): Behavioral Counseling: Cases and Techniques." New York: Holt, Rinehart and Winston. Part 1, pp. 7–18, Intro.
41. Brownell KD (1982): Obesity: Understanding and treating a serious prevalent and refractory disorder. J Consult Clin Psychol 50:820–840.
42. Foreyt JP, Mitchell RE, Garner DT, Gee M, Scott LW, Gotto AM (1982): Behavioral treatment of obesity: Results and limitations. Behav Ther 13:153–163.
43. Stunkard AJ, Penick SB (1979): Behavior modification in the treatment of obesity: The problem of maintaining weight loss. Archives of General Psychiatry, 36, 810–816.
44. Wadden, TA, personal communication, Department of Psychiatry, University of Pennsylvania, 133 S. 36th St. Philadelphia, PA 19104.
45. LeBow, MD, 1981, *Weight control: The behavioral strategies.* New York: Wiley, 1981.
46. Stuart RB (1979): Weight loss and beyond: Are they taking it off and keeping it off? In Davidson PO (ed): "Behavioral Medicine: Techniques for Promoting Life-style Change." New York: Brunner/Mazel. pp. 151–194.
47. Wilson GT (1980): Behavioral therapy for obesity. In Stunkard AJ (ed), "Obesity" Philadelphia: Saunders, (pp 325–344).
48. Wilson GT, Brownell KD (1980): Behavior therapy for obesity: An evaluation of treatment outcome. Adv Behav Res Ther 3:49–86.
49. Jeffery RW, Wing RR, Stunkard AJ (1978): Behavioral treatment of obesity: State of the art in 1976. Behav Ther 6:189–199.
50. Marlatt GA, Gordon JR (eds): (1985): "Relapse Prevention: Maintenance Strategies in Addictive Behavior Change. New York: Guilford.
51. Brownell KD, Marlatt GA, Lichtenstein E, Wilson GT (1986): Understanding and preventing relapse. 41:7, 765–782.
52. Hughes GH, Hymowitz N, Ockene J, Simon N, Vogt TH (1981): The Multiple Risk Factor Intervention Trial (MRFIT) V> Intervention on smoking. Prev Med 10:476–500.

53. Lichtenstein E (1982): The smoking problem: A behavioral perspective. J Consult Clin Psychol 50:804–819.
54. Wilson GT (1985): Psychologist prognostic factors in the treatment of obesity. In Hirsch J, Van Itallie TB (eds), ''Recent Advances in Obesity Research,'' vol. 4. London: Libbey, pp 301–311.

Section B:

EMERGING ISSUES RELATED TO CALCIUM INTAKE

Nutritional Factors in Hypertension
© *1990 Alan R. Liss, Inc., pages 99–106*

| 7 | # Calcium Metabolism in Health and Chronic Diseases: An Overview
David A. McCarron, M.D. |

INTRODUCTION

This review will serve as an introduction to the specific topics considered in this monograph's presentation of issues surrounding calcium metabolism in health and various disease states. Over the past five years, no macronutrient has received more attention than dietary calcium. Abnormalities of calcium metabolism and/or an epidemiological link to reduced dietary calcium intake have been associated with a variety of common, chronic medical disorders. These include osteoporosis, hypertension, type II diabetes, morbid obesity, colon cancer, and alcohol-related heart disease. While these associations are intriguing, in most cases the observations remain preliminary in nature and the pathophysiological mechanisms are unknown. We will consider in detail the specifics of the epidemiological link between lower dietary calcium intake and hypertension, the blood pressure response to increasing calcium intake, the physiology of intestinal calcium absorption, and active cellular calcium transport in the following chapters. These topics should be considered against the backdrop of increasing evidence that dietary calcium and the regulation of overall calcium metabolism may be a pathological link in the genesis of common, chronic diseases in humans. The recent evidence supporting that postulate will serve as the focus of this introduction to the symposium.

From the Division of Nephrology and Hypertension, Department of Medicine, Oregon Health Sciences University, Portland, OR 97201.

EPIDEMIOLOGY: DIETARY CALCIUM AND
CHRONIC DISORDERS

Public health measures relating diet to health promotion have emphasized reductions in specific nutrients. Lower sodium chloride intake has been promoted for reducing the risk of hypertensive heart disease [1], while lower cholesterol intake has been encouraged as a means of reducing atherosclerotic heart disease [2]. In the face of this emphasis on dietary excesses contributing to common chronic diseases, evidence from a large number and variety of epidemiologic studies indicates that correction of dietary calcium deficiency may hold substantial potential to reduce the occurrence of a variety of common medical disorders, particularly in the aging population. While there remains controversy surrounding the question of whether sodium or cholesterol intake is truly excessive in the general population, little doubt exists that in most developed societies the daily intake of calcium from the diet is well below minimum requirements in many humans [3]. This point has been particularly emphasized for female subjects; however, for many males, it is equally true. Estimates project that 30–50% of males over age 35 regularly consume less than the current recommended daily allowance (RDA) of calcium (800–1000 mg). For both males and females this figure worsens with age, and for black individuals the percentage of subjects underconsuming calcium is even greater.

There is general agreement that lifelong restriction of dietary calcium intake, particularly during adolescence and early adulthood in women, contributes to the later development of osteoporosis [4]. The emergence of serious bone mineral loss after menopause has its greatest effects in those women who fail to develop optimal bone mass earlier in life. It has been more difficult to document that increasing dietary calcium intake will retard or reverse this process in older women [5]. There is agreement, nevertheless, that women should endeavor to maintain a minimum of 1000 to 1400 mg of calcium intake daily as a preventive measure against excessive bone mineral loss postmenopause [6]. With the exception of alcoholics, there is little evidence that men face the same risk of osteoporosis as women [7].

Hypertension has been identified as another chronic disorder that is linked to failure to consume an adequate level of dietary calcium [8]. Twenty-five epidemiologic studies have examined this association, and all but one have verified its existence [9]. These surveys have principally come from the United States, although three have sampled European populations. In the United States, the age range has spanned from infancy (1 month) to 75 years. It has been demonstrated in both sexes and in a variety of racial and ethnic groups. The association has been shown to be independent, in part, of exercise, alcohol intake, smoking history, level of education, other nutrients, and body-mass index. There are some important interactions between dietary calcium and several of these variables [10], and these will be discussed below. In at least three of the reports, a threshold for the emergence of an increased risk of hypertension in the population under observation was noted [11–13]. The threshold rests at 400 to 600 mg per day. At levels below this, the risk of becoming hypertensive may increase 25 to 40%. This association is more evident in men under the age of 50 and women older than 55–60 years [13]. Several of the reports have linked low dietary calcium consumption to high risk groups that include the elderly [14], blacks [15,16], pregnant women [17], and oriental males [18]. The results of several of these dietary analyses have linked dietary calcium's effect on blood pressure to postulated effects of other dietary constituents on cardiovascular disease, including sodium, potassium, magnesium, phosphorus, and protein. One recent study has verified this cardioprotective effect in a prospective assessment of the relationship of diet to chronic diseases [12].

Dietary calcium intake has also been associated with body-mass index in two of these epidemiological surveys [13,19]. While it would normally be assumed that nutrient consumption is typically higher in the obese individual, this is not the case for dietary calcium. Independent relationships have been reported between lower calcium intake and increased body-mass index. This association appears to be not only inverse but also linear. It can be demonstrated in both normotensive and hypertensive populations.

An association between dietary calcium and colon cancer has been noted in one large survey [20]. The combined exposure to increasing levels of dietary calcium and exposure to increasing levels of dietary calcium and vitamin D was linked to at least a 60% decrease in the probability of developing colon cancer. Similar to the dietary calcium intake and arterial pressure relationship, the colon cancer association appears to be nonlinear, with a threshold of approximately 300 to 400 mg per day. Below that level, the risk of developing colon cancer increased dramatically over a 20-year period of observation.

No epidemiological study to date has demonstrated an association between the level of dietary calcium and the emergence of alcohol abuse. Three studies, however, have reported that dietary calcium consumption is related to alcohol's effects on blood pressure [19,21,22]. Many surveys have confirmed that as alcohol ingestion increases in a population, the risk of developing hypertension climbs steeply [19,23,24]. In the three studies noted previously, an interaction between alcohol and calcium in the diet was reported. In each case, the findings suggested that maintenance of a higher level of calcium in the diet was protective against the development of alcohol-associated hypertension.

CLINICAL AND EXPERIMENTAL EVIDENCE OF CALCIUM'S EFFECTS ON CHRONIC DISORDERS

For osteoporosis, it is generally agreed that maintaining a higher level of calcium in the diet than is currently consumed by females in the United States will afford some protection against postmenopausal bone mineral loss. This effect is greater where concurrent estrogen use is present [5]. In addition, factors that are thought to modify adversely the bioavailability of dietary calcium are also associated with an increased risk of developing osteoporosis. These include lack of exercise, higher dietary protein intake, and glucocorticol use. In a naturally occurring model of accelerated bone mineral loss, we have recently demonstrated that failure to maintain an adequate level of dietary calcium will reduce bone calcium content significantly [25].

The relationship of calcium metabolism to high blood pressure, while still controversial [26], has been clarified substantially in the past few years. Besides the epidemiological data cited above, clinical and experimental evidence supports the hypothesis that failure to maintain adequate calcium homeostasis increases arterial pressure [8]. In humans with hypertension, a variety of abnormal biochemical parameters consistent with impaired calcium metabolism have been reported [8,9]. In several experimental models of high blood pressure, virtually identical findings have been reported and extended to include evidence of abnormal cellular calcium metabolism in not only vascular tissue but several other cell lines as well [27].

The link between these alterations in calcium metabolism and the development of hypertension in the laboratory has been strengthened by the arterial pressure responses to supplemental dietary calcium in these animal models. In each model, supplementation of the diet with calcium results in either the prevention of the experimental hypertension or the reversal of the hypertension if it is already established [9]. More importantly, the arterial pressure response in humans to adding calcium to their daily regimen is similar. Using dietary sources or various calcium salts, the blood pressure of both hypertensive and normotensive subjects has been demonstrated to decrease when 500 to 1500 mg additional calcium is ingested daily [9]. In the published, controlled intervention trials, approximately 35 to 45% of the subjects have been responsive, demonstrating at least a 5 to 10 mmHg reduction in pressure compared to placebo. Consistent with the results of other dietary interventions to lower blood pressure, some individuals (estimated at 10 to 15%) have higher blood pressures during the calcium phase than when they are on placebo. Men and women are both responsive, although males may be slightly more so. Significant reductions in both systolic and diastolic blood pressures have been detected. Young and older individuals with elevated blood pressures have been sensitive. On average, systolic blood pressure has dropped 7 to 10 mmHg and diastolic pressure 3 to 7 mmHg in the various trials.

The possible association of type II diabetes and abnormal calcium metabolism is based on more limited clinical and experimental observations [28,29]. Specifically, humans with type II or adult-onset diabetes manifest several abnormalities of calcium homeostasis that suggest the presence of calcium deficiency. More recently, the coexistence of type II diabetes and disordered calcium metabolism has been described in one of the experimental models of hypertension [30]. Whether an intervention to reverse the deranged homeostasis will modify the course of the impaired carbohydrate metabolism has not been addressed in either humans or experimental models.

Several alterations of calcium metabolism have been characterized in the morbidly obese [31,32]. They parallel many of the findings in type II diabetics and hypertensives and may reflect the concordance of these common disorders in the same subjects [33]. Our laboratory has recently demonstrated in a rodent model that manipulating dietary calcium intake will favorably influence body-fat composition [34]. As calcium consumption increases, body fat decreases and lean body mass rises.

For colon cancer, the data are limited. In one human trial, individuals at high risk of developing colon cancer were shown to favorably improve the histology of precancerous polyps when 1250 mg of additional calcium was consumed for two to three months [35]. The application of this finding has not been pursued on a larger scale in high-risk population or considered for other malignancies.

There is no research evidence that increasing dietary calcium will alter the clinical course of alcohol abuse, although that possibility is suggested by the epidemiological findings noted above and the reports of metabolic evidence of calcium deficiency in chronic alcoholics. It is especially noteworthy that clinically significant osteoporosis, which is unusual in males, is relatively common in the male alcoholic [7].

SUMMARY

The concept that failure to maintain adequate dietary calcium intake contributes to the emergence of a number of common medical disorders that afflict the aging population in our society, while intriguing, remains entirely speculative at this time. As the information that I have briefly summarized here suggests, there is reason to pursue that possibility through scientific investigation. We need to explore more thoroughly the epidemiological associations in order to provide additional clues as to where and how to proceed in clinical studies, as well as in the laboratory. The recent experience with the epidemiological identification of an association between hypertension and calcium intake, which is summarized in one of the articles in this monograph, can serve as an example of the potential value of further work in this area.

Likewise, our need to better understand the factors that influence intestinal calcium absorption will increase. Simply assuming that increasing daily calcium intake alone without carefully considering how the ingested mineral's intestinal transport may be modified could possibly impair or even prevent the intended clinical outcome. The review of intestinal calcium absorption provided by Dr. Drüeke will serve as an excellent starting point for those clinicians and researchers who are interested.

The expansive growth of cellular physiology and molecular biology as it relates to calcium's effects on normal cell function must be thoroughly understood. If there is a common link through calcium metabolism that accounts for the overlap in some individuals of more than one of the common medical disorders speculated upon in this chapter, exposition of that mechanism will come from research at the subcellular level. The information summarized by Dr. Vincenzi provides a useful review of several aspects of calcium's unique role in regulating cell function.

Ultimately, additional research in this broad area should result in improved therapy and prevention of some portion of these disorders in populations at high risk. Dr. Sowers's assessment of calcium metabolism in blacks is an important example of the preventive aspects of our endeavors to increase calcium intake in populations where intake is well below the current RDA, which, as described above, may contribute to a variety of chronic disorders that exact a terrible toll in premature morbidity and mortality.

REFERENCES

1. Joint National Committee (1988): The 1988 report of the Joint National Committee on detection, evaluation, and treatment of high blood pressure. Arch Intern Med 184:1023–1038.
2. National Cholesterol Education Program Adult Treatment Panel. Cholesterol treatment recommendations for adults. Bethesda MD, National Heart, Lung and Blood Institute, 1987.
3. Sempos C, Cooper R, Kovar MG, Johnson C, Drizd T, Yetley E (1986): Dietary calcium and blood pressure in National Health and Nutrition Examination Surveys I and II. Hypertension 8:1067–1074.
4. Freudenheim JL, Johnson NE, Smith EL (1986): Relationship between usual nutrient intake and bone-mineral content of women 35–65 years of age: longitudinal and cross-sectional analysis. Am J Clin Nutr 44:863–876.
5. Riis B, Thomsen K, Christiansen C (1987): Does calcium supplementation prevent postmenopausal bone loss? N Engl J Med 316:173–177.
6. Spencer H, Kramer L (1986): NIH consensus conference: osteoporosis. Factors contributing to osteoporosis. J Nutr 116:316–319.
7. Bikle DD, Genant HK, Cann C, Recker RR, Halloran BP, Strewler GJ (1985): Bone disease in alcohol abuse. Ann Intern Med 103:42–48.

8. McCarron DA, Morris CD (1987): The calcium deficiency hypothesis of hypertension. Ann Intern Med 107:919–922.

9. McCarron DA (1989): Calcium metabolism and hypertension. Kidney Int 35:717–736.

10. Morris CD, McCarron DA (1987): Dietary calcium intake in hypertension. Hypertension 10:350–351.

11. Joffres MR, Reed DM, Yano K (1987): Relationship of magnesium intake and other dietary factors to blood pressure: the Honolulu heart study. Am J Clin Nutr 45:469–475.

12. Witteman JCM, Willett WC, Stampfer MJ, Colditz GA, Sacks BR, Rosner B, Speizer FE, Hennekens CH (1987): Dietary calcium and magnesium and hypertension: a prospective study. Circulation 76:iv–35.

13. McCarron DA, Morris CD, Henry HJ, Stanton JL (1984): Blood pressure and nutrient intake in the United States. Science 224:1392–1398.

14. Harlan WR, Hull AL, Schmouder RL, Landis JR, Larkin FA, Thompson FE (1984): High blood pressure in older americans. Hypertension 6:802–809.

15. Langford HG (1987): Dietary sodium, potassium, and calcium in black hypertensive subjects. J Clin Hypertens 3:36S–42S.

16. Liebman M, Chopin LF, Carter E, Clark AJ, Disney GW, Hegsted M, Kenney MA, Kirmani ZA, Koonce KL, Korslund MK, Moak SW, McCoy H, Stallings SF, Wakefield T (1986): Factors related to blood pressure in a biracial adolescent female population. Hypertension 8:843–850.

17. Belizän JM, Villar J (1980): The relationship between calcium intake and edema-, proteinuria-, and hypertension-gestosis: an hypothesis. Am J Clin Nutr 33:2202–2210.

18. Reed D, McGee D, Yamo K, Hankin J (1985): Diet, blood pressure and multicollinearity. Hypertension 7:405–411.

19. Kromhout D, Bosachieter EB, Coulander G (1985): Potassium, calcium, alcohol intake and blood pressure: the Zutphen Study. Am J Clin Nutr 41:1299–1304.

20. Garland C, Shekelle RB, Barrett-Connor E, Criqui MH, Rossof AH, Paul O (1985): Dietary vitamin D and calcium and risk of colorectal cancer: a 19-year prospective study in men. Lancet, Feb:307–309.

21. Gruchow HW, Sobocinski KA, Barboriak JJ (1985): Alcohol, nutrient intake and hypertension in US adults. JAMA 253:1567–1570.

22. Criqui MH, Langer RD, Reed DM (1988): Dietary alcohol, calcium and potassium: effects on blood pressure. CVD Epidemiol News 43:30.

23. Gordon T, Kannel WB (1983): Drinking and its relation to smoking, BP, blood lipids and uric acid: the Framingham study. Arch Intern Med 143:1366–1374.

24. MacMahon SW, Norton RN (1986): Alcohol and hypertension: implications for prevention and treatment. Ann Intern Med 105:124–126.

25. Metz JA, Karanja N, McCarron DA (1988): Bone density comparison in two hypertensive strains: effects of dietary sodium. Clin Res 36:A139.

26. Kaplan NM, Meese RB (1986): The calcium deficiency hypothesis of hypertension: a critique. Ann Intern Med 105:947–955.

27. Young EW, Bukoski RD, McCarron DA (1988): Calcium metabolism in experimental hypertension. Proc Soc Exp Biol Med 187:123–141.

28. Levin ME, Boisseau VC, Avioli LV (1975): Effects of diabetes mellitus on bone mass in juvenile and adult-onset diabetes. N Engl J Med 294:241–245.

29. Heath H III, Lambert PW, Service FJ, Arnaud SB (1979): Calcium homeostasis in diabetes mellitus. J Clin Endocrinol Metab 49:462–466.

30. Mondon CE, Reaven GM (1988): Evidence of abnormalities of insulin metabolism in rats with spontaneous hypertension. Metabolism 37:303–305.

31. Bell NH, Epstein S, Greene A, Shary J, Oeximann MJ, Shaw S (1985): Evidence for alteration of the vitamin D-endocrine system in obese subjects. J Clin Invest 76:370–373.

32. Andersen T, McNair P, Fogh-Andersen N, Nielsen TT, Hyldstrup L, Transbøl I (1986): Increased parathyroid hormone as a consequence of changed complex binding of plasma calcium in morbid obesity. Metabolism 35:147–151.

33. Modan M, Halkin H, Almog S, Lusky A, Eshkol A, Shefi M, Shitrit A, Fuchs Z (1985): Hyperinsulinemia: a link between hypertension obesity and glucose intolerance. J Clin Invest 75:809–817.

34. Metz JA, Karanja N, Torok J, McCarron DA (1988): Modification of total body fat in spontaneously hypertensive rats and Wistar-Kyoto rats by dietary calcium and sodium. Am J Hypertens 1:58–60.

35. Lipkin M, Newmark H (1985): Effect of added dietary calcium on colonic epithelial-cell proliferation in subjects at high risk for familial colonic cancer. N Engl J Med 313: 1381–1384.

Nutritional Factors in Hypertension
© *1990 Alan R. Liss, Inc., pages 107–130*

8 | Calcium Metabolism in Hypertension

Eric W. Young, M.D.
Richard D. Bukoski, Ph.D.
David A. McCarron, M.D.

INTRODUCTION

A diverse body of research data has emerged recently that suggests an association between hypertension and altered calcium metabolism [1]. While the full significance of this association is still evolving, it has opened a promising area in hypertension research at the epidemiologic, clinical, whole-animal, and cellular levels [1].

Three principal lines of evidence link calcium metabolism and hypertension. First, analysis of several large epidemiologic data bases suggest an inverse relationship between blood pressure and dietary calcium intake. Similarly, the prevalence of hypertension appears to be inversely correlated with calcium intake. Second, alterations in systemic and cellular calcium metabolism that may contribute to or reflect calcium deficiency have been described in both experimental and human hypertension. Specifically, both intestinal calcium malabsorption and renal calcium wasting have been reported. Third, supplemental oral calcium lowers blood pressure both in hypertensive animals and in humans. This finding is consistent with the correction of a calcium deficit resulting in a favorable arterial pressure response. Thus, both reduced levels of dietary calcium intake and abnormal systemic calcium handling are associated with hypertension.

To integrate these two fundamental observations, it has been proposed that

From the Department of Medicine, Division of Nephrology and Hypertension, Department of Physiology, Oregon Health Sciences University, 3181 S.W. Sam Jackson Park Road, Portland, OR 97201.

some forms of hypertension are a manifestation of low calcium intake in an individual with a compromised ability to conserve calcium. Depending on the circumstances, one or both of these conditions may be sufficient to cause or contribute to elevated systemic pressure. Altered calcium metabolism may play a role in essential or genetic hypertension, as well as in secondary forms of hypertension such as primary aldosteronism and renal vascular disease. This chapter, which is based upon an earlier review [2], will focus on systemic and cellular calcium metabolism in experimental and human essential hypertension after a brief discussion of the epidemiologic data.

EPIDEMIOLOGY OF CALCIUM AND BLOOD PRESSURE

Population-based studies of calcium and hypertension were initially prompted by a report that untreated hypertensive subjects appeared to have a renal calcium leak despite elevated serum parathyroid hormone [3]. A pilot population survey that looked at the relationship between dietary calcium intake and blood pressure [4] and a subsequent larger analysis [5] of the first Health and Nutrition Examination Survey database (HANES-I) uncovered a significant, inverse relationship between dietary calcium intake and blood pressure. This relationship has been confirmed by other investigators using the HANES as well as other population databases, including diverse ethnic groups and geographical regions [6–21]. While these epidemiologic surveys have been consistent in showing a relationship between low dietary calcium intake and hypertension, they do not establish causality. However, they have stimulated investigation into systemic and cellular calcium metabolism in both humans and experimental hypertension. These efforts have identified a number of alterations in calcium metabolism associated with human and experimental high blood pressure.

SYSTEMIC CALCIUM METABOLISM IN HYPERTENSION

Hypertensive animals and humans demonstrate several distinct alterations in calcium (Ca^{2+}) metabolism at the systemic level that may affect Ca^{2+} balance. The specific systemic manifestations of abnormal calcium metabolism in either experimental or human hypertension include: low serum-ionized Ca^{2+} concentrations, elevated serum parathyroid hormone (PTH) levels, inappropriate renal calcium losses, and alterations of intestinal calcium absorption and $1,25(OH)_2$ vitamin D_3 metabolism. Ultimately, these disturbances affect total body and bone Ca^{2+} balance. Calcium metabolism in the laboratory has been best characterized in the spontaneously hypertensive rat (SHR), although substantial data also exist for several other experimental models of hypertension and for human essential hypertension. Blood pressure and calcium handling, like other physiologic processes, change as the hypertensive animal matures, and also vary by gender of the animal. Therefore, the age and sex of the animals in the SHR studies discussed below are emphasized for a more clear understanding of the evolution of the abnormalities of calcium metabolism that are associated with arterial hypertension.

Normal Calcium Metabolism

When discussing differences in Ca^{2+} handling between hypertensive and normotensive animals or humans, it must be realized that both intracellular and extracellular Ca^{2+} levels are tightly regulated by the PTH-vitamin D_3 axis. Small differences in markers of calcium homeostasis may reflect a significant metabolic defect, which may be minimized by compensatory regulatory processes. Until the cellular basis for abnormal Ca^{2+} metabolism in hypertension is understood, it will be difficult to determine if the various hormonal and functional alterations are primary or compensatory in origin.

Serum Calcium

A low serum-ionized calcium concentration ($[Ca^{2+}]_s$) in the SHR, relative to its normotensive control, the Wistar-Kyoto rat (WKY), was found at 5 and 13 weeks of age in female rats [22] and at 8, 10, 16, 24, 33, 40, and 45 weeks in males [23–25]. On average, $[Ca^{2+}]_s$ in WKY exceeded that in SHR by approximately 0.15 mEq/L. Whether the specimens were taken from fasted or fed animals was generally not specified. Wright also found decreased $[Ca^{2+}]_s$ in SHR as compared with normotensive Sprague-Dawley rats [26]. By contrast, Lau et al. reported higher postabsorptive $[Ca^{2+}]_s$ in 25-week-old female SHR and no difference in fasting $[Ca^{2+}]_s$ between 26-week-old female SHR and WKY [27]. However, these experiments were performed on parathyroidectomized rats. The same authors found that fasting plasma ultrafilterable Ca^{2+} was lower in parathyroid-intact, 23-week-old female SHR. After parathyroidectomy, there was no difference in plasma ultrafilterable Ca^{2+} between SHR and WKY. Plasma ultrafilterable Ca^{2+} includes ionized calcium (~80%) as well as complexed, nonprotein bound Ca^{2+} (~20%). A reasonable interpretation of these studies is that $[Ca^{2+}]_s$ is decreased in the parathyroid-intact SHR but that the difference from WKY is obliterated by removal of the parathyroid glands. More recently, Lau et al. [28] reported no difference in $[Ca^{2+}]_s$ between 25-day-old parathyroid-intact SHR and WKY of both genders. Thus, it appears that $[Ca^{2+}]_s$ is initially normal in SHR but falls as the arterial pressure rises. The uninephrectomized DOCA-salt hypertensive rat also exhibits low $[Ca^{2+}]_s$, while the one-kidney, one-clip and two-kidney, one-clip rat models of renovascular hypertension do not [22].

Total serum calcium is not altered in SHR in any consistent direction. The combination of low $[Ca^{2+}]_s$ and normal total serum calcium implies an increase in serum protein-bound Ca^{2+} in SHR. Direct measurements in humans with essential hypertension confirm decreased serum-ionized, complexed, and ultrafilterable Ca^{2+} and increased protein-bound Ca^{2+} [29]. Other investigators have also reported low $[Ca^{2+}]_s$ in human essential hypertension [30,31] and in patients with primary aldosteronism [32].

Parathyroid Hormone and Urinary Cyclic AMP

Typically, serum parathyroid hormone (PTH) levels are elevated in the SHR, presumably as a secondary response to the low $[Ca^{2+}]_s$. Stern et al. [24] found that carboxy-terminal PTH was detectable in 43% of 6-week-old and 55% of 10-week-old male SHR, whereas all of the WKY of the same ages had undetectable C-terminal PTH levels. In this study, $[Ca^{2+}]_s$ was significantly lower in 10-week-old SHR than in the WKY. Bindels et al. (23) also found elevated immunoreactive PTH and decreased $[Ca^{2+}]_s$ in 8-week-old SHR, although another assay for intact PTH showed no difference between SHR and WKY. McCarron et al. [30] found that amino-terminal PTH was significantly elevated in male SHR at 18, 24, and 29 weeks of age. A C-terminal assay also revealed higher serum PTH in the SHR at 29 weeks. Again $[Ca^{2+}]_s$ was significantly lower in the SHR at these ages. A mid-molecule PTH assay failed to detect a difference between the SHR and WKY [33]. Recently, SHR were shown to have hyperplasia of the parathyroid glands, providing anatomical evidence for chronic stimulation of their parathyroid glands [34]. Elevated serum PTH concentration has also been reported in humans with essential hypertension [3,35,36] and with primary aldosteronism [32].

While serum PTH levels may be appropriately elevated in the SHR in response to decreased $[Ca^{2+}]_s$, end-organ responsiveness may be abnormal. Basal nephrogenous cyclic AMP is lower in 11- to 17-week-old male SHR than in WKY (37). Total urinary cyclic AMP has been reported to be decreased [27,37] or normal [38] in 13- to 16-week-male SHR. Normal or decreased urinary cyclic AMP in the face of elevated serum PTH is consistent with renal unresponsiveness to the peptide hormone. Further evidence for reduced renal response to PTH in the SHR includes elevated $U_{Ca}V$ in the setting of higher PTH levels [25] and a subnormal increment in $1,25(OH)_2$ vitamin D production in response to PTH infusion [39]. Furthermore, PTH infusion caused a smaller increment in $[Ca^{2+}]_s$ in 13-week-old male SHR than in WKY [40]. In vitro studies also suggest abnormal cyclic AMP generation as adenylate cyclase activity of isolated renal membranes from 5- and 16-week-old SHR was reduced in response to PGE_2, although the response to other stimuli and basal activity were normal [41]. In sum, the SHR's ability to compensate for a low $[Ca^{2+}]_s$ by renal mechanisms is compromised. In contrast, in human essential hypertension, urinary cyclic AMP is appropriately elevated [35] in response to elevated serum PTH that has been reported in this patient population [3,35].

Calcium Excretion

Urinary calcium excretion is increased in the mature SHR, although there is disagreement as to whether this reflects primary intestinal hyperabsorption or a primary renal calcium leak. Preadolescent 24-hour urinary calcium has been variously reported as decreased [23,28], not different [25,27,40,42], and increased [27,42,43]. As the SHR reaches maturity, its urinary calcium excretion exceeds that of the WKY. Longitudinal studies indicate that hypercalciuria develops in male SHR by 17 weeks of age and in females by 25 to 26 weeks. McCarron et al. [25] reported significantly increased calcium excretion in 17-, 22-, 28-, and 43-week-old male SHR with concurrently low $[Ca^{2+}]_s$ and elevated serum PTH concentrations. The hypercalciuria was interpreted to reflect a renal calcium leak. That is, the kidneys of maturing and mature SHR fail to normally reabsorb calcium despite a lower filtered calcium load and a higher level of serum PTH. The latter should stimulate renal Ca^{2+} reabsorption. On a low-Ca^{2+} diet, hypercalciuria was enhanced in 18- to 20-week-old male SHR [44], providing further evidence for a renal leak.

In female SHR, Lau et al. found higher 24-hour calcium excretion beginning at 25 weeks age [27]. Parathyroidectomy enhanced hypercalciuria in the 25-week-old female SHR. Urinary calcium excretion after fasting was decreased in 23-week-old females [27] and in 8- to 14-week old males [38]. The relevance of these findings, however, is questionable, as 24-hour urinary calcium excretion is increased only in older SHR. Nonetheless, based on low fasting calcium excretion and normal urinary cyclic AMP (PTH was not measured), the 24-hour hypercalciuria was felt to result from increased intestinal calcium absorption [27] and not from diminished renal tubular calcium reabsorption.

The critical distinction between absorptive and renal hypercalciuria remains unsettled because of differences in sex and age of animals used in various studies and in actual measurements of calcium balance. A further complication arises because the SHR may have defective calcium metabolism involving several organs, which prevents anticipated compensatory responses. Expected findings with a primary renal calcium leak include: fasting hypercalciuria and ionized hypocalcemia; elevated serum PTH, urinary cyclic AMP, and serum $1,25(OH)_2D_3$; parathyroid hyperplasia; and negative (or neutral) calcium balance relative to WKY [45]. In short, renal hypercalciuria is consistent with whole-animal calcium deficiency in SHR. Absorptive hypercalciuria predicts normal fasting urinary and serum-ionized Ca, suppressed parathyroid function and gland size, and positive (or neutral) Ca balance relative to WKY [45]. Pure absorptive hypercalciuria therefore indicates calcium surfeit rather than deficit. This will be further addressed after discussion of Ca absorption, vitamin D metabolism, and Ca balance in this animal model.

Hypercalciuria is also found in the uninephrectomized, DOC-treated rat model in response to feeding sodium chloride but not sodium bicarbonate [46]. In this model, hypercalciuria precedes the onset of hypertension. Similarly, urinary calcium excretion is increased in the Dahl salt-sensitive hypertensive rat [47] and in the Milan rat strain of spontaneous hypertension [48] compared to their respective normotensive controls. Hypercalciuria appeared to be on a renal basis in both the DOC and Milan hypertensive strains. Thus, hypercalciuria is common to several forms of experimental hypertension. A possible explanation for the hypercalciuria may be decreased renal adenylate cyclase response to PTH as described for Dahl salt-sensitive and DOC-NaCl hypertensive rats [49]. The Milan hypertensive strain also exhibits decreased renal Ca^{2+}-ATPase activity [50]. Either end-organ response failure to PTH's actions or reduced Ca^{2+} pump activity could account for the renal leak of calcium.

Increased urinary calcium excretion has also been found in human essential hypertension [3,51]. Basal 24-hour urinary calcium excretion was higher in hypertensive than in normotensive control subjects, despite comparable urinary sodium excretion [3,35]. Acute calcium infusion produced higher urinary calcium excretion for a given filtered calcium load in humans [35,52].

Calcium Absorption

Intestinal calcium transport and net absorption have been studied by several techniques with seemingly conflicting results. The in vitro everted duodenal sac preparation estimates net active and passive transfer of radiolabeled Ca^{2+} from the mucosal to the serosal surface. Several investigators have found no difference in duodenal Ca^{2+} absorption in 5- and 10-week-old male SHR [24,53], increased absorption in 12-week-old male SHR [53], and decreased absorption in 5- and 12-week-old male SHR [54]. Schedl et al. [55] recently found lower intestinal calcium transport in SHR obtained from three different breeders as compared with their normotensive controls. Similarly, in vivo techniques for measuring duodenal radioactive Ca^{2+} transfer have indicated both increased absorption in 12-week-old male [53] and 50-week-old female SHR [27] as well as decreased absorption in 12-week-old male SHR [54]. These particular discrepancies cannot be readily explained by differences in experimental technique or diet.

Another in vitro approach has been to employ the modified Ussing chamber technique. This method provides a direct measurement of active Ca^{2+} flux across isolated intestinal segments. Ca^{2+} flux driven by the electrochemical gradient is eliminated by voltage clamping the preparation and by exposing the mucosal and serosal membrane surfaces to the same concentration of Ca^{2+}. Using this technique, the unidirectional mucosal-to-serosal Ca^{2+} flux was significantly reduced in 12- to 14-week-old male SHR when compared to the WKY [56,57]. Ca^{2+} secretion (serosal-to-mucosal flux) was not different between SHR and WKY. Thus, net duodenal Ca^{2+} flux across the isolated duodenal segment was reduced in the adolescent SHR [56,57]. By contrast, Ussing studies on 24- [57] and 35-week-old [58] male animals revealed no difference between SHR and WKY in unidirectional and net Ca^{2+} flux across duodenum and colon on a normal Ca^{2+} diet, although duodenal flux was reduced in 24-week-old SHR maintained on a low Ca^{2+} diet [57].

Isolated duodenal enterocytes provide another technique for assessment of Ca^{2+} metabolism in intestinal epithelium. Influx of radiolabeled [45]Ca using this technique was decreased in enterocytes isolated from the proximal duodenum of 12- to 14-week and 28- to 32-week-old male SHR as compared with age-matched WKY [59,60]. Also, [45]Ca efflux was decreased in enterocytes from 12- to 14-week-old SHR [61]. While isolated cellular flux data do not measure actual transmucosal Ca^{2+} flux, they do indicate that one step of intestinal Ca^{2+} transport is reduced in growing as well as mature male SHR.

Because in vitro and segmental in vivo techniques may not fully account for differences in paracellular and segmental intestinal calcium absorption, measurements of whole-animal Ca^{2+} absorption have been attempted. Stern et al. [24] performed balance studies on male SHR and WKY from 6 to 10 weeks of age and reported no significant difference in cumulative Ca intake and mean daily urinary and fecal calcium excretion. Over the four-week balance study, SHR retained 180 ± 15 mg Ca^{2+} as compared with 218 ± 24 mg Ca^{2+} in WKY. Cumulative Ca absorption calculated from these authors' measurements of Ca intake and fecal excretion was 89.2 mg for SHR and 169 mg for WKY over the last 2 weeks of the balance period, suggesting a trend for reduced Ca^{2+} absorption and less cumulative balance in the growing male SHR. Similarly, Lau et al. [27] found reduced fractional Ca^{2+} absorption and a trend for reduced absolute Ca^{2+} absorption and Ca^{2+} retention in 10-week-old male SHR over a 6-day balance study. By contrast, Bindels et al. [23] found no difference in Ca^{2+} absorption in 6- and 8-week-old male SHR, and Hsu et al. [38] reported increased Ca^{2+} absorption in 13- to 16-week-old male SHR based upon increased urinary Ca^{2+} excretion following an oral load of either cold or radiolabeled Ca^{2+}. Increased Ca^{2+} absorption was also found in balance experiments performed on

3½-week-old prehypertensive male and female SHR (28) and in mature hypertensive 25- and 50-week-old female SHR [27]. In general, these data from several laboratories using different diets indicate that male SHR malabsorb Ca^{2+} during maturation and the developmental phase of their hypertension. Calcium malabsorption becomes less apparent as the SHR ages. In very early life, male SHR may exhibit increased calcium absorption. Female SHR hyperabsorb Ca^{2+} at all ages studied (3.5, 25, and 50 weeks). There is currently no explanation for these differences between sexes. The findings in the female remain to be confirmed in other laboratories. Unfortunately, the balance technique for measuring Ca^{2+} absorption in small animals cannot accurately measure small differences in Ca^{2+} absorption and is subject to error, especially if urine or feces become contaminated with uneaten food.

Bone Mineralization

Since bone is the largest store of Ca^{2+} in the body, bone mineralization should provide a more accurate index of whole animal Ca^{2+} balance. Bone mineralization reflects net Ca^{2+} retention as determined by intestinal absorption and urinary excretion of calcium and the net action of PTH and $1,25(OH)_2D_3$, as well as other Ca^{2+} regulating hormones. In male SHR, bone Ca^{2+} content (mg Ca/gm fat-free dry weight) was not different from WKY at 6 and 18 weeks of age [23,38], but was significantly decreased at 23 [57] and 54 [62] weeks of age. Similarly, ash weight/volume, and ash weight/dry weight of the femoral bone were unchanged in 6-week-old male SHR [23], but were reduced in 26-week-old male SHR [63]. Bone cortical thickness was also reduced in the 26-week-old animal. By contrast, a study of hydralazine-treated female SHR reported increased fractional bone mass and Ca^{2+} density at one year of age [27].

Thus, bone Ca^{2+} is normal in early life in male SHR, but is less than that observed in the WKY as the animals reach late adolescence and early adulthood. Reduced bone Ca^{2+} content in SHR is consistent with reduced Ca^{2+} retention over time. These differences are not apparent in the female SHR. To date, Ca^{2+} absorption, balance, and bone status have not been measured in other experimental models or in human hypertension.

Vitamin D Metabolism

Vitamin D metabolism is abnormal in the SHR, partially accounting for the decreased intestinal Ca absorption. Altered vitamin D regulation may also be involved in the increased renal excretion of Ca^{2+} and altered cellular Ca^{2+} metabolism associated with hypertension. While serum levels of $1,25(OH)_2D$ are reported to be elevated [23,28] or unchanged [24,54,64,65] in young male SHR from 3 to 13 weeks of age, a number of laboratories have detected low basal serum $1,25(OH)_2D$ concentration in SHR as early as 11 weeks of age [34,39,57,65,66]. That is, low serum $1,25(OH)_2D$ levels are found just as the SHR is developing hypertension and Ca^{2+} malabsorption. Low or even normal serum $1,25(OH)_2D$ levels are clearly inappropriate, since the SHR have low $[Ca^{2+}]_s$, low serum phosphorus [23,43], and elevated PTH. Serum 25(OH)D tends to be elevated in the SHR, indicating that vitamin D intake or substrate availability is not compromised and therefore cannot account for the inappropriately low $1,25(OH)_2D$ [54,65,67]. Additional evidence for altered vitamin D metabolism in the SHR is indicated by subnormal increments in serum $1,25(OH)_2D_3$ in response to PTH administration [39,64], cyclic AMP stimulation [39], and phosphate depletion [39,66]. The response of serum $1,25(OH)_2D$ to a low Ca^{2+} diet has been reported to be both decreased [57] and normal [65] in the SHR. The low basal and PTH-stimulated serum $1,25(OH)_2D$ in SHR can be accounted for by a reduced production rate, since metabolic clearance of $1,25(OH)_2D$ is not different in SHR and WKY [33]. Still more evidence for abnormal vitamin D metabolism is found in the observation that SHR, but not WKY, develop hypocalcemia and low serum $1,25(OH)_2D$ when placed on a vitamin D–deficient diet between the ages of 4 and 13 weeks [67]. Serum 25(OH)D falls to undetectable levels in both groups, although only WKY are able to maintain $1,25(OH)_2D$ and Ca^{2+} homeostasis.

The mechanism of abnormal $1,25(OH)_2D$ production in the SHR is unknown. Intrinsic 1-α-hydroxylase enzyme activity of isolated renal mitochondria appears to be normal or even enhanced [64]. Cyclic AMP generation is involved in PTH-stimulation of $1,25(OH)_2D$ production [68]. Although urinary cyclic AMP generation is decreased in SHR, cyclic AMP infusion results in a smaller increment in serum $1,25(OH)_2D_3$ in SHR than in WKY, suggesting that an additional defect is involved [39]. Increased intracellular or mitochondrial concentration of Ca^{2+}, inorganic phosphate, or hydrogen ion could possibly suppress activity of the 1-α-hydroxylase enzyme in renal proximal tubules, as these are postulated regulators of the enzyme. There is some evidence for systemic acidosis [69] and phosphate retention [23,70] in SHR. Intracellular ionic status has not been measured. Cytosolic free Ca^{2+} is elevated in some cells of the SHR (see below), but preliminary reports indicate unchanged or low levels in renal proximal tubules [71,72].

Although some studies have suggested that SHR display intestinal resistance to the effects of $1,25(OH)_2D_3$ [53,54], more recent work demonstrates normal [57] or increased [73] intestinal response to the hormone. Lucas et al. [57] found that Ca^{2+} flux across isolated duodenal segments measured by Ussing apparatus is normalized in SHR when they are given supplemental $1,25(OH)_2D_3$. Similarly, the calcemic response to systemic PTH infusion is blunted in SHR and is normalized when the animals are given $1,25(OH)_2D_3$

[40]. Thus, it appears that the defective vitamin D metabolism reported in the SHR is of functional importance.

Vitamin D metabolism may also be altered in human hypertension. Resnick et al. [74] reported high serum $1,25(OH)_2D$ in patients with low-renin hypertension and low-serum $1,25(OH)_2D$ in patients with high-renin hypertension. For each renin group, serum $1,25(OH)_2D_3$ varied inversely with serum ionized Ca^{2+}, although the appropriateness of the response was not assessed quantitatively. These investigators hypothesize that $1,25(OH)_2D_3$ is an important factor in the mediation of low-renin hypertension.

Integrated View of Ca^{2+} Metabolism in SHR

In view of the above-described alterations in Ca^{2+} metabolism in experimental hypertension, it is worthwhile to attempt a synthesis of the various observations into a unified view of calcium status. While a parallel exists between Ca^{2+} metabolism in the SHR and human essential hypertension, it is too early to extrapolate the laboratory findings to the human situation. Differences between SHR and WKY are more likely to be found when the animals are on a relatively low Ca^{2+} diet. Male SHR have been studied most extensively and are known to develop earlier and higher elevations of blood pressure than female SHR; therefore, most comments apply to the male.

The major discrepancies in the literature concern the issue of intestinal Ca^{2+} transport and absorption. Nonetheless, many investigators find evidence for reduced Ca^{2+} absorption in adolescent SHR. As the animals age, the difference between SHR and WKY diminishes. Basal serum $1,25(OH)_2D$ is elevated in the very young SHR, but ultimately decreases as the animal matures. Nonetheless, the reduced serum-ionized Ca^{2+} and elevated serum PTH levels at a very young age suggest that net calcium retention is less in the SHR compared to the WKY. However, gross Ca^{2+} depletion is not manifest until adulthood when decreased bone Ca^{2+} content is found. Finally, hypercalciuria appears in late adolescence just prior to the time when a measurable reduction in bone mineralization occurs. While the cause of the increased urinary calcium has been disputed [25,27,38], the predominant finding of reduced or normal calcium absorption and reduced bone calcium argues strongly against an intestinal hyperabsorption for the excessive urinary calcium excretion. Furthermore, the findings of low serum-ionized Ca^{2+} concentration, elevated PTH levels, and parathyroid hyperplasia [34] in SHR essentially fulfills the criteria for renal hypercalciuria (cf. above). Urinary cyclic AMP and serum $1,25(OH)_2D$ are not elevated, as one would predict in the setting of renal hypercalciuria. This suggests that a defect exists in the cellular systems that control their production and release by the kidney. In female SHR, $[Ca^{2+}]_s$ falls early, but hypercalciuria occurs later than in males for unclear reasons. More extensive longitudinal studies of systemic Ca^{2+} metabolism in both genders of experimental models of hypertension would be valuable.

Effect of Calcium Loading

Although provocative, the systemic alterations in Ca^{2+} handling are of uncertain relevance to hypertension. Since Ca^{2+} is the critical intracellular mediator of vascular smooth muscle contraction, an attractive explanation for abnormal systemic Ca^{2+} metabolism invokes an intrinsic abnormality of pan-cellular Ca^{2+} metabolism that results in elevated vascular tone and altered intestinal and renal Ca^{2+} handling. An important link between the existence of abnormal systemic Ca^{2+} metabolism and the development of hypertension is the observation that dietary Ca^{2+} supplementation lowers blood pressure in SHR [25,42,56,75,76], other experimental models of hypertension [77–79], and in human essential hypertension [51,80].

The mechanism of the antihypertensive effect of dietary Ca^{2+} is not known. Calcium may decrease sympathetic nerve activity as judged by circulating catecholamines or the systemic response to stress [81]. Some investigators have found that dietary Ca^{2+} promotes natriuresis [42], although others have not [75,76], and supplemental dietary Na appears to augment the hypotensive effect of Ca [56]. The effect of dietary Ca^{2+} has also been ascribed to phosphate depletion [76]. Increasing oral phosphate intake, however, lowers blood pressure, a result that would not be predicted by the phosphate-depletion hypothesis [82,83]. Ca^{2+} may also lower blood pressure by virtue of its effect on PTH, vitamin D metabolites, or other hormones such as calcitonin gene-related peptide [84], all of which may have acute and chronic vascular actions. Finally, dietary calcium may favorably modulate a defect in cellular Ca^{2+} handling, leading to normalization of systemic Ca^{2+} handling and blood pressure. For example, a high-calcium diet caused increased Ca^{2+} influx in enterocytes isolated from SHR and reduced Ca^{2+} influx in enterocytes isolated from WKY; the net result was that Ca^{2+} influx became the same in SHR and WKY as compared with a normal Ca^{2+} diet [60]. Whatever the mechanism by which Ca^{2+} lowers blood pressure, an understanding of the cellular processes behind abnormal systemic Ca^{2+} metabolism is essential.

CELLULAR CALCIUM METABOLISM

The questions of whether organ-level disturbances in Ca^{2+} metabolism in humans with essential hypertension and in the SHR reflect a primary alteration in cellular calcium metabolism and whether these cellular defects play a causal role in chronically elevated blood pressure are pertinent. One would predict that Ca^{2+} metabolism of vascular smooth muscle is abnormal in the hypertensive state if indeed this cell type is involved in a primary fashion in the pathogenesis of the disease as opposed to playing a passive role. Direct investigation in the human situation has been limited, mostly as a result of difficulties encountered in obtaining appropriate tissue samples and cell types. As a result, the majority of information has been drawn from studies on formed elements of the blood derived from humans with essential hypertension or using vascular tissue isolated from animal models of hypertension.

Vascular Smooth Muscle

A widely espoused hypothesis accounting for hypertension of vascular origin is that there is a defect in the ability of the vascular smooth muscle cell to maintain normal levels of intracellular Ca^{2+}, principally through a depressed control system. Cellular Ca^{2+} metabolism has been studied using a variety of techniques, including measurement of flux of ^{45}Ca into intact tissues and isolated membrane preparations, enzymatic analysis of pumps or carriers believed to play a role in the regulation of intracellular levels of Ca^{2+}, and more recently, the use of intracellular indicators to assess free levels of intracellular Ca^{2+}. Studies of vascular smooth muscle isolated from the SHR that have examined ^{45}Ca influx into whole tissue have shown either an increase [85], no change [86], or a decrease in influx [87]. These results, of course, are dependent upon the age of the animal, the time course over which influx was determined, and the method of defining intracellular vs. extracellular ^{45}Ca. Only limited conclusions about specific pools of Ca^{2+} or binding sites can be drawn from this type of investigation. While early studies focused on conduit arteries, Cauvin et al. [88,89] have recently examined unidirectional influx of ^{45}Ca into mesenteric resistance vessels of the SHR and observed enhanced influx of Ca^{2+} under both basal and norepinephrine-stimulated conditions. These studies derive support from the finding of Mulvany et al. [90] that resistance arteries of the mesenteric bed have an increased sensitivity to extracellular Ca^{2+}. These results, in addition to the observations that Ca^{2+} channel blockers have a greater blood pressure lowering effect and vasodilator action in essential hypertension than in control subjects, have been interpreted to indicate that the cell membrane of vascular smooth muscle is more permeable to Ca^{2+} in the hypertensive state [91–93]. In fact, a recent report by Rusch and Hermsmeyer [94] demonstrated an increased distribution of the L-type channel in the vascular smooth muscle cell of the SHR when compared to the WKY.

Studies of Ca^{2+} transport by isolated membrane fractions of vascular smooth muscle show a consistent trend that suggests a depressed ability of the smooth muscle cell membrane to actively transport Ca^{2+}. When ATP-supported Ca^{2+} uptake was measured in microsomal fractions of aorta isolated from the SHR [85,95,96] or from cell membrane enriched fractions of mesenteric arteries of the SHR [97,98], uptake was attenuated compared with fractions isolated from normotensive controls. It is possible that this decrease in uptake is a reflection of an abnormal cell membrane Mg^{2+}/Ca^{2+}-ATPase pump.

Perhaps a more rigorous approach would combine Ca^{2+} uptake studies using isolated membrane vesicles with kinetic analyses of the purified Mg^{2+}/Ca^{2+}-ATPase. While this enzyme has been purified from both aortic muscle of the cow [99] and smooth muscle of the pig antrum [100,101], it has not been possible to purify it from vascular smooth muscle of the rat. Therefore, the enzyme has not been well characterized in experimental hypertension. On the other hand, Mg^{2+}/Ca^{2+}-ATPase isolated from other smooth muscle systems has been shown to be activated by calmodulin and have a requirement for Mg^{2+} as well as Ca^{2+} and ATP, and is similar to membrane-associated Ca^{2+}-ATPase from other organ systems, i.e., skeletal and cardiac muscle [102]. Therefore, it may be inferred that the enzyme is similar in the various smooth muscle types, but knowledge of potential differences in either its activity or activation characteristics in the setting of elevated pressure does not exist.

In addition to the Ca^{2+}-ATPase transport system, the Na^+-Ca^{2+} exchange carrier may also play a role in the regulation of intracellular Ca^{2+}. At least two groups have detected the presence of this carrier in cell-membrane-enriched fractions of vascular smooth muscle [103,104]. In the former study, a comparison of Na^+-Ca^{2+} exchange activity of cell-membrane-enriched fractions of mesenteric arteries of the SHR and WKY was carried out and no differences were detected.

Besides these transport systems that are directly involved in Ca^{2+} transport, the Na^+,K^+-ATPase/sodium pump system is believed to play a role in the regulation of intracellular Ca^{2+} levels by its electrogenic contribution to the membrane potential and thus an indirect effect on potential-operated Ca^{2+} channels [105]. The sodium pump also regulates levels of intracellular sodium and may help set the level of, and interface with, intracellular Ca^{2+} via the Na^+-Ca^{2+} exchange mechanism discussed above. To date, several models of experimental hypertension show depressed sodium pump function when assessed indirectly via either ^{86}Rb uptake [106] or potassium-induced relaxation of isolated vessels [107]. However, when the number of pump sites in aorta of SHR and WKY was determined using ^3H-ouabain binding, no differences were detected [108], indicating that the pumps may be different physiologically but perhaps not enzymatically or biochemically.

In addition to the sodium pump, a second transport system that may be linked to Ca^{2+} regulation via alterations in intracellular Na^+ is the

Na^+-H^+ exchanger. This carrier has been identified in membrane preparations of vascular smooth muscle [109] and is activated by the diacyl glycerol arm of the phosphotidylinositol pathway [110]. While it has been suggested to provide a major Na^+ influx pathway [111], it has not been studied to date in vascular smooth muscle of the SHR or its normotensive control.

Given this discussion of the various systems involved in the regulation of intracellular Ca^{2+} levels, the primary question remains as to whether intracellular Ca^{2+} concentration is altered under basal or stimulated conditions. Studies using ^{45}Ca allow some estimation of influx rates and total exchangeable Ca^{2+} binding sites, but do not allow delineation between bound and free Ca^{2+}. A recent advancement in this area has been the application of the intracellular Ca^{2+} dyes Quin-2, Fura-2, and Indo-1 to both smooth muscle and formed elements. Several studies have examined intracellular Ca^{2+} levels in vascular smooth muscle during hypertension using a Ca^{2+}-sensitive dye. Nabika et al. [112] examined monolayer of cells grown on coverstrips and found no differences in intracellular Ca^{2+} between the SHR and WKY. In contrast, Sugiyama et al. [113] examined both primary and passaged smooth muscle cells and found that intracellular Ca^{2+} was higher in vascular smooth muscle cells of 12-week-old SHR. In considering these disparate findings, differences in loading efficiencies and the effects of cell dispersion techniques or culture conditions on subsequently observed differences or similarities of the response between cells from hypertensive and normotensive animals must be evaluated. More recently, Bukoski et al. [114] reported that intracellular free Ca^{2+} levels are not different in intact mesenteric arteries of SHR compared to WKY.

Platelets

In addition to vascular smooth muscle of hypertensive animal models, Ca^{2+} metabolism has also been studied in formed elements of the blood of humans with essential hypertension and SHR, with the expectation that differences observed in these cell types are reflections of differences also present in vascular smooth muscle cells or that the same (humoral or pharmacologic) factors that induce changes in formed elements also impinge on vascular smooth muscle cells and resistance vessels. To date, platelets have been most extensively studied, primarily because of the relative ease and quantity in which they are obtained as well as their similarity to vascular smooth muscle in terms of second messenger responses [115].

Several groups have identified an increase in the intracellular levels of Ca^{2+} in platelets derived from people with essential hypertension using

Quin-2 [116–120] and more recently Fura-2 [121] as an intracellular indicator. Erne et al. [116] and Le Quan Sang et al. [119] observed a positive relationship between blood pressure and intracellular Ca^{2+} concentration. Furthermore, Erne et al. [116] observed a fall in intracellular Ca^{2+} when blood pressure was lowered with antihypertensive therapy. This may be interpreted to indicate that either the humoral profile of the plasma compartment was altered to provide for a lowering of intracellular Ca^{2+} in the platelet or that the platelets themselves were affected in a manner parallel to that of the vascular smooth muscle. It should also be considered that "shear stress" experienced by the platelets during their course through resistance vessels and capillaries may vary with mean arterial pressure and thus be a direct cause of elevated intracellular Ca^{2+} as has been reported for red blood cells [122]. If this is the case, then the measurement of intracellular Ca^{2+} in platelets as a marker for changes in vascular smooth muscle Ca^{2+} metabolism in the face of increased arterial pressure is limited.

In addition to intracellular Ca^{2+} concentration, platelet Ca^{2+}-ATPase has been examined in essential hypertension. Overall Ca^{2+}-ATPase activity was greater in platelets of hypertensive subjects, while calmodulin stimulated the ATPase to a lesser extent than in controls [123]. While these results do not readily explain the elevated levels of intracellular Ca^{2+} reported in platelets, these investigators suggest that the elevated Ca^{2+}-ATPase capacity reflects a negative feedback control mechanism by which the cell protects itself from a Ca^{2+} overload.

Erythrocytes

In addition to platelets, erythrocytes have been studied in human and experimental hypertension, primarily because of the major role that the cell membrane Ca^{2+}-ATPase plays in regulating red cell Ca^{2+} concentration and the ease of obtaining samples. Postnov et al. [124] examined Na^+ permeability and Ca^{2+} binding capacity (defined as the pool removable by incubation with EDTA), and found that Na^+ flux was elevated while extracellular Ca^{2+} binding capacity was depressed during hypertension. Furthermore, intracellular Ca^{2+} was observed to have an inhibitory action on Na^+-K^+-ATPase function in red cells in essential hypertension, and this has been interpreted to reflect a depressed inner-cell-membrane binding capacity. In a later study, Postnov et al. [125] reaffirmed the findings of depressed binding of Ca^{2+} to outer membranes of red cell ghosts as well as studying the Ca^{2+}-ATPase activity of erythrocytes obtained from humans with essential hypertension. They found that upon depletion of the preparation of calmodulin, no differences in Ca^{2+}-ATPase activity were observed between hypertensive subjects and normotensive controls. Upon readdition of calmodulin, however, the erythrocyte Ca^{2+}-ATPase from hypertensive subjects was stimulated to a lesser degree, while there was no difference in the distribution of calmodulin in red cells of the two groups. These data, and the report of a biochemical characterization of calmodulin isolated from the brains of SHR and WKY which showed no differences in the affinity of the activation protein for Ca^{2+} or in its ability to stimulate phosphodiesterase activity [126], have been interpreted to indicate that a defect in the enzyme that is specific to the enzyme's capacity to be stimulated by calmodulin may be present in hypertension.

Vincenzi et al. [127] examined Ca^{2+}-ATPase activity of red cells of hypertensive and normotensive humans. The results showed that basal Ca^{2+}-ATPase activity, defined as ATPase activity resistant to inhibition by the calmodulin inhibitor trifluoroperazine, was depressed in those with high blood pressure, while maximal stimulated activity was not different. While these data do not agree with those of Postnov et al. [128], a study by Olorunsogo et al. [129] reported that maximum red cell Ca^{2+}-ATPase activity was depressed with hypertension, but activation by calmodulin was normal. Further work is needed to clarify these issues.

Other Formed Elements

In addition to platelets and red cells, intracellular Ca^{2+} levels have also been examined in neutrophils by Lew et al. [130] and no differences were observed between normotensive and hypertensive individuals. These authors concluded that not all cell types demonstrate elevated levels of intracellular Ca^{2+} during hypertension. Bruschi et al. [131] used lymphocytes from the SHR and observed a higher concentration of free intracellular Ca^{2+} compared with cells derived from control, but the level of intracellular Ca^{2+} was not influenced by alterations in extracellular Ca^{2+} or by the addition of ouabain or catecholamines. These latter, negative findings suggest that a problem existed in the in vitro preparation of the cells these investigators employed [131].

Summary of Cellular Ca^{2+} Metabolism

Based on our review of cellular Ca^{2+} metabolism in hypertension, vascular smooth muscle in experimental hypertension may exhibit changes in basic mechanisms of Ca^{2+} regulation. Much additional experimental work is required before the picture will be complete. It may well be that changes in Ca^{2+} metabolism of the formed elements reflects altered physiology of the organism in terms of responses to humoral factors, but the degree to which they reflect similar changes in vascular muscle remains to be answered and may be unrelated to the pathogenesis of elevated peripheral vascular resistance and arterial pressure.

CONCLUSION

Calcium metabolism is altered in hypertension at both the whole-animal and cellular levels. Furthermore, dietary Ca^{2+} deficiency is associated with human hypertension at the epidemiological level, and oral Ca^{2+} supplementation lowers blood pressure in human and experimental hypertension. In this chapter, we have presented the integrated view that a constellation of systemic abnormalities of Ca^{2+} metabolism in hypertension results in inefficient Ca^{2+} conservation and relative Ca^{2+} deficiency. Furthermore, the cellular findings in hypertension suggest increased cell membrane Ca^{2+} permeability and a compromised ability of the cell to remove or sequester intracellular Ca^{2+}. Paradoxically, this leads to increased intracellular free Ca^{2+} in the face of reduced extracellular Ca^{2+} levels. Unfortunately, most of the whole-animal and cellular work has been carried out using different tissues. Nevertheless, it is reasonable to hypothesize that abnormal Ca^{2+} handling in the cell is ultimately reflected at the organ and whole-animal level so that alterations in vascular smooth muscle, intestine, kidney, and erythrocytes are due to the same underlying defect manifested in many cell lines. The primary cell defect may involve the membrane imbedded Ca^{2+}-ATPase pump [60], an intrinsic membrane-binding protein [132], a cell membrane Ca^{2+} channel, or some other process.

If an underlying cellular defect in Ca^{2+} metabolism exists in some forms of hypertension, what is the link with elevated blood pressure? While altered Ca^{2+} metabolism in hypertension may be an epiphenomenon of some other metabolic process that is primarily responsible for the elevated blood pressure, a more central role for altered Ca^{2+} metabolism in hypertension is suggested by the myriad of defects that have been reported. The issue will remain unsettled, however, until the molecular bases for abnormal calcium and vascular homeostasis in hypertension are established. Understanding of calcium metabolism and blood pressure regulation in hypertension, whether as shared or separate mechanisms, will be a challenging and likely rewarding area of future clinical and basic research.

ACKNOWLEDGMENTS

Funds for the preparation of this paper were provided by the Dairy Bureau of Canada. Some of the original research cited in this paper was supported by grants from the MJ Murdock Charitable Trust, the Oregon Affiliate of the American Heart Association, the American Heart Association, the National Dairy Board, and administered in cooperation with the National Dairy Council, the National Kidney Foundation, and a General Clinical Research Center award from the U.S. Public Health Service.

REFERENCES

1. McCarron DA (1989): Calcium metabolism and hypertension. Kidney Int 35:717–736.
2. Young EW, Bukoski RD, McCarron DA (1988): Calcium metabolism in essential hypertension. Proc Soc Exp Biol Med 187:123–141.
3. McCarron DA, Pingree PA, Rubin RJ, Gaucher SM, Molitch M, Krutzik S (1980): Enhanced parathyroid function in essential hypertension: a homeostatic response to a urinary calcium leak. Hypertension 2:162–168.
4. McCarron DA, Morris CD, Cole C (1982): Dietary calcium in human hypertension. Science; 217:267–269.
5. McCarron DA, Morris CD, Henry HJ, Stanton JL (1984): Blood pressure and nutrient intake in the United States. Science 224:1392–1398.
6. Harlan WR, Hull AL, Schmouder RL, Landis JR, Thompson RE, Larkin FA (1984): Blood pressure and nutrition in adults. The National Health and Nutrition Examination Survey. Am J Epidemiol 120:17–28.
7. Harlan WR, Hull AL, Schmouder RL, Landis JR, Larkin FA, Thompson FE (1984): High blood pressure in older Americans. The First National Health and Nutrition Examination Survey. Hypertension 6:802–809.
8. Joffres MR, Reed DM, Yano K. Relationship of magnesium intake and other dietary factors to blood pressure: the Honolulu Heart Study. Am J Clin Nutr 45:469–475.
9. Gruchow HW, Sobocinski KA, Barboriak JJ (1988): Calcium intake and the relationship of dietary sodium and potassium to blood pressure. Am J Clin Nutr 48:1463–1470.
10. Harlan WR, Landis JR, Schmouder RL, Goldstein NG, Harlan LC (1985): Blood lead and blood pressure: relationship in the adolescent and adult US population. JAMA 253:530–534.
11. Garcia-Palmieri MR, Costas R Jr, Cruz-Vidal M, Sorlie PD, Tillotson J, Havlik RJ (1984): Milk consumption, calcium intake, and decreased hypertension in Puerto Rico. Puerto Rico Heart Health Program Study. Hypertension 6:322–328.
12. Ackley S, Barrett-Connor E, Suarez L (1983): Dairy products, calcium, and blood pressure. Am J Clin Nutr 38:457–461.
13. Reed D, McGee D, Yano K, Hankin J (1985): Diet, blood pressure, and multicollinearity. Hypertension 7:405–410.
14. Nichaman M, Shekelle R, Paul O (1984): Diet, alcohol, and blood pressure in the Western Electric Study. Am J Epidemiol 120:469–470.
15. Kromhout D, Bosschieter EB, Coulander CL (1985): Potassium, calcium, alcohol intake and blood pressure: the Zutphen Study. Am J Clin Nutr 41:1299–1304.
16. Yamamoto M, Kuller L (1985): Calcium and elevated blood pressure—further evidence from the Three-Area Stroke Mortality Study. Am J Epidemiol 122:512.
17. Yamamoto ME, Kuller LH (1985): Does dietary calcium influence blood pressure? Evidence from the Three-Area Stroke Mortality Study. Circulation 72:111–116.
18. Caggiula AW, Milas NC, McKenzie JM, Sugars C (1986): Nutrient intake and blood pressure in the multiple risk factor intervention trial. (Abstract). American Heart Association Council on Cardiovascular Epidemiology. p 155.
19. Kok FJ, Vandenbroucke JP, Van Der Heide-Wessel C, Van Der Heide RM (1986): Dietary sodium, calcium, and potassium, and blood pressure. Am J Epidemiol 123:1043–1048.
20. Liebman M, Chopin LF, Carter E, et al. (1986): Factors related to blood pressue in a biracial adolescent female population. Hypertension 8:843–850.
21. Trevisan M (1986): Relationship between total and varied sources of dietary calcium intake and blood pressure. Am J Epidemiol 124:507.

22. Wright GL, Rankin GO (1982): Concentrations of ionic and total calcium in plasma of four models of hypertension. Am J Physiol 243:H365–H370.

23. Bindels RJM, Van Den Brock LAM, Jongen MJM, Hackeng WHL, Lowik CWGM, Van Os CH (1987): Increased plasma calcitonin levels in young spontaneously hypertensive rats: role in disturbed phosphate homeostasis. Pflügers Arch 408:395–400.

24. Stern N, Lee DBN, Silis V, et al. (1984): Effects of high calcium intake on blood pressure and calcium metabolism in young SHR. Hypertension 6:639–646.

25. McCarron DA, Yung NN, Ugoretz BA, Krutzik S (1981): Disturbances of calcium metabolism in the spontaneously hypertensive rat. Hypertension 3:I162–I167.

26. Wright GL, Toraason MA, Barbe JS, Crouse W (1980): The concentrations of ionic and total calcium in plasma of the spontaneously hypertensive rat. Can J Physiol Pharmacol 58:1494–1499.

27. Lau K, Zikos D, Spirnak J, Eby B (1984): Evidence for an intestinal mechanism in hypercalciuria of spontaneously hypertensive rats. Postgrad Med 247:E625–E633.

28. Lau K, Langman CB, Gafter U, Dudeja PK, Brasitus TA (1986): Increased calcium abosrption in prehypertensive spontaneously hypertensive rats. Role of serum 1,25-dihydroxyvitamin D3 levels and intestinal brush border membrane fluidity. J Clin Invest 78:1083–1090.

29. Folsom AR, Smith CL, Prineas RJ, Grimm RH Jr (1986): Serum calcium fractions in essential hypertensive and matched normotensive subjects. Hypertension 8:11–15.

30. McCarron DA (1982): Low serum concentrations of ionized calcium in patients with hypertension. N Engl J Med 307:226–228.

31. Resnick LM, Laragh JH, Sealey JE, Alderman MH (1983): Divalent cations in essential hypertension. Relations between serum ionized calcium, magnesium, and plasma renin activity. N Engl J Med 309:888–891.

32. Resnick LM, Laragh JH (1985): Calcium metabolism and parathyroid function in primary aldosteronism. Am J Med 78:385–390.

33. Young EW, Hsu CH, Patel S, Simpson RU, Komanicky P (1987): Metabolic degradation and synthesis of calcitriol in spontaneously hypertensive rat. Am J Physiol 252:E778–E782.

34. Merke J, Slotkowski A, Mann H, Lucas PH, Drueke T, Ritz E (1987): Abnormal 1,25(OH)$_2$D$_3$ receptor status in genetically hypertensive rats. Kidney Int 31:303.

35. Strazzullo P, Nunziata V, Cirillo M, et al. (1983): Abnormalities of calcium metabolism in essential hypertension. Clin Sci 65:137–141.

36. Grobbee DE, Hofman A (1986): Effect of calcium supplementation on diastolic blood pressure in young people with mild hypertension. Lancet ii:703–706.

37. McCarron DA (1983): Impaired nephrogenous cAMP response in the spontaneously hypertensive rat. Kidney Int 23:106.

38. Hsu CH, Chen P-S, Smith DE, Yang C-S (1986): Pathogenesis of hypercalciuria in spontaneously hypertensive rats. Min Electrol Metab 12:130–141.

39. Young EW, Patel SR, Hsu CH (1986): Plasma 1,25(OH)$_2$D$_3$ response to parathyroid hormone, cyclic adenosine monophosphate, and phosphorus depletion in the spontaneously hypertensive rat. J Lab Clin Med 108:562–566.

40. Hsu CH, Patel S, Young EW (1987): Calcemic response to parathyroid hormone in spontaneously hypertensive rats: role of calcitriol. J Lab Clin Med 110:682–689.

41. Umemura S, Smyth D, Pettinger W (1984): Defective renal adenylate cyclase response to prostaglandin E$_2$ in spontaneously hypertensive rats. Kidney Int 25:338.

42. Ayachi S (1979): Increased dietary calcium lowers blood pressure in the spontaneously hypertensive rat. Metabolism 28:1234–1238.

43. Hsu CH, Chen PS, Caldwell RM (1984): Renal phosphate excretion in spontaneously hypertensive and normotensive Wistar Kyoto rats. Kidney Int 25:789–795.

44. Grady JR, Dorow J, McCarron DA (1983): Urinary calcium excretion and cAMP response of the spontaneously hypertensive rat to Ca^{2+} deprivation. Clin Res 31:330A.

45. Coe FL, Favusm MJ (1986): Disorders of stone formation. In Brenner BM, Rector FC (eds): "The Kidney." pp 1403–1422.

46. Kurtz TW, Morris RC Jr (1985): Dietary chloride as a determinant of disordered calcium metabolism in salt-dependent hypertension. Life Sci 36:921–929.

47. Umemura S, Smyth DD, Nicar M, Rapp JP, Pettinger WA (1986): Altered calcium homeostasis in Dahl hypertensive rats: physiological and biochemical studies. J Hypertens 4:19–26.

48. Cirillo M, Galletti F, Corrado MF, Strazzullo P (1986): Disturbances of renal and erythrocyte calcium handling in rats of the Milan hypertensive strain. J Hypertens 4:443–449.

49. Umemura S, Smyth DD, Pettinger WA (1986): Renal adenylate cyclase in Dahl and DOC-Na hypertensive rats: defective response to parathyroid hormone with calcium leak. J Hypertens 4:s291–s293.

50. Bianchi G, Ferrari P, Salvati P, et al. (1986): A renal abnormality in the Milan hypertensive strain of rats and in humans predisposed to essential hypertension. J Hypertens 4:s33–s36.

51. McCarron DA, Morris CD (1985): Blood pressure response to oral calcium in persons with mild to moderate hypertension. Ann Intern Med 103:825–831.

52. Ellison DH, Shneidman R, Morris C, McCarron DA (1986): Effects of calcium infusion on blood pressure in hypertensive and normotensive humans. Hypertension 8:497–505.

53. Toraason MA, Wright GL (1981): Transport of calcium by duodenum of the spontaneously hypertensive rat. Am J Physiol 241:G344–G347.

54. Schedl HP, Miller DL, Pape JM, Horst RL, Wilson HD (1984): Calcium and sodium transport and vitamin D metabolism in the spontaneously hypertensive rat. J Clin Invest 73:980–986.

55. Schedl HP, Wilson HD, Horst RL (1988): Calcium transport and vitamin D in three breeds of spontaneously hypertensive rats. Hypertension 12:310–316.

56. McCarron DA, Lucas PA, Shneidman RJ, Lacour B, Drueke T (1985): Blood pressure development of the spontaneously hypertensive rat after concurrent manipulations of dietary Ca^{2+} and Na^+: relation to intestinal Ca^{2+} fluxes. J Clin Invest 76:1147–1154.

57. Lucas PA, Brown RC, Drueke T, Lacour B, Metz JA, McCarron DA (1986): Abnormal vitamin D metabolism, intestinal calcium transport, and bone calcium status in the spontaneously hypertensive rat compared with its genetic control. J Clin Invest 78:221–227.

58. Gafter U, Kathpalia S, Zikos D, Lau K (1986): Ca fluxes across duodenum and colon of spontaneously hypertensive rats: effect of $1,25(OH)_2D_3$. Am J Physiol 251:F278–F282.

59. Roullet CM, Young EW, Roullet J-B, Drueke T, McCarron DA (1989): Calcium uptake by duodenal enterocytes isolated from young and mature SHR and WKY rats. Am J Physiol (in press).

60. Roullet C, Drueke T, McCarron D (1987): Ca^{2+} influx of SHRs' isolated enterocytes: normalization by dietary Ca^{2+}. Kidney Int 31:308.

61. Lucas PA, Roullet CM, Duchambon P, Lacour B, Dang P, McCarron DA, Drueke T (1989): Decreased duodenal enterocyte calcium flux rates in spontaneously hypertensive rats. Am J Hypertens 2:86–92.

62. Metz JA, Karanja N, McCarron DA (1989): Characterization of bone calcium, magnesium, and density in the spontaneously hypertensive rat: differential effects of dietary calcium and sodium. Am J Clin Nutr (in press).
63. Izawa Y, Sagara K, Kadota T, Makita T (1985): Bone disorders in spontaneously hypertensive rat. Calcif Tissue Int 37:605–607.
64. Kawashima H (1986): Altered vitamin D metabolism in the kidney of the spontaneously hypertensive rat. Biochem J 237:893–897.
65. Schedl HP, Miller DL, Horst RL, Wilson HD, Natarajan K, Conway T (1986): Intestinal calcium transport in the spontaneously hypertensive rat: response to calcium depletion. Am J Physiol 250:G412–G419.
66. Kurtz TW, Portale AA, Morris RC Jr (1986): Evidence for a difference in vitamin D metabolism between spontaneously hypertensive and Wistar-Kyoto rats. Hypertension 8:1015–1020.
67. Hsu CH, Yang C-S, Patel SR, Stevens MG (1987): Calcium and vitamin D metabolism in spontaneously hypertensive rats. Am J Physiol 253:F712–F718.
68. Horiuchi N, Suda T, Takahashi H, Shimazawa E, Ogata E (1977): In vivo evidence for the intermediary role of 3′,5′-cyclic AMP in parathyroid hormone-induced stimulation of 1a,25-dihydroxyvitamin D₃ synthesis in rats. Endocrinology 101:969–974.
69. Lucas PA, Lacour B, McCarron DA, Drueke T (1987): Disturbance of acid-base balance in the young spontaneously hypertensive rat. Clin Sci 73:211–215.
70. Eby B, Salvi D, Lau K (1986): Pathophysiology and consequence of reduced PO₄ excretion in the spontaneously hypertensive rat. "Proc First Ann Mtg Am Soc Hypertens." New York: American Society of Hypertension, p 29A.
71. Jacobs WR, Brazy PC, Mandel LJ (1987): Fura 2 measurements of intracellular free calcium in renal cortical tubules from SHR and WKY rats. Kidney Int 31:350.
72. Llibre J, LaPointe MS, Batlle DC (1988): Free cytosolic calcium in renal proximal tubules from the spontaneously hypertensive rat. Hypertension 12:399–404.
73. Gafter U, Eby B, Martin C, Lau K (1986): Response of spontaneously hypertensive rats to 1,25(OH)₂D₃ in vivo. Kidney Int 30:497–512.
74. Resnick LM, Muller FB, Laragh JH (1986): Calcium regulating hormones in essential hypertension. Relation to plasma renin activity and sodium metabolism. Ann Intern Med 105:649–654.
75. Kageyama Y, Suzuki H, Hayashi K, Saurta T (1986): Effects of calcium loading on blood pressure in spontaneously hypertensive rats: attenuation of the vascular reactivity. Clin Exp Hypertens A8:355–370.
76. Lau K, Chen S, Eby B (1984): Evidence for the role of PO₄ deficiency in antihypertensive action of a high-Ca diet. Am J Physiol 246:H324–H331.
77. Kageyama Y, Suzuki H, Arima K, Saruta T (1987): Oral calcium treatment lowers blood pressure in renovascular hypertensive rats by suppressing the renin-angiotensin system. Hypertension 10:375–382.
78. Kageyama Y, Suzuki H, Arima K, Kondo K, Saruta T (1987): Effects of calcium loading in DOCA-salt hypertensive rats. Jpn Circ J 51:1315–1324.
79. Benedetti RG (1986): Dietary calcium supplementation lowers blood pressure in renovascular hypertension without severe phosphorus depletion. J Hypertens 4 (suppl 5): s565.
80. Luft FC, Aronoff GR, Sloan RS, Fineberg NS, Weinberger MH (1986): Short-term augmented calcium intake has no effect on sodium homeostasis. Clin Pharmacol Ther 39:414–419.
81. Hatton DC, Huie PE, Muntzel MS, Metz JA, McCarron DA (1987): Stress-induced blood pressure responses in SHR: effect of dietary calcium. Am J Physiol 252:R48–R54.

82. Jones MR, Ghaffari F, Tomerson BW, Clemens RA (1986): Hypotensive effect of a high calcium diet in the Wistar rat. Min Electrol Metab 12:85–91.

83. Bindels RJM, Van Den Brock LAM, Hillebrand SJW, Wokke JMP (1987): A high phosphate diet lowers blood pressure in spontaneously hypertensive rats. Hypertension 9:96–102.

84. Goodman EC, Iversen LL (1986): Calcitonin gene-related peptide: novel neuropeptide. Life Sci 38:2169–2178.

85. Bhalla RC, Webb RC, Singh D, Ashley T, Brock T (1978): Calcium fluxes, calcium binding, and adenosine cyclic 3'5'-monophosphate-dependent protein kinase activity in the aorta of spontaneously hypertensive and Kyoto Wistar normotensive rats. Mol Pharmacol 14:468–477.

86. Zsoter TT, Wolchinsky C, Henein NF, Ho LC (1977): Calcium kinetics in the aorta of spontaneously hyeprtensive rats. Cardiovasc Res 11:353–357.

87. Shibata S, Kuchii M, Taniguchi T (1975): Calcium flux and binding in the aortic smooth muscle from the spontaneously hypertensive rat. Blood Vess 12:279–289.

88. Cauvin C, Van Breemen C (1985): Altered ^{45}Ca fluxes in isolated mesenteric resistance vessels from SHR. Fed Proc 44:1008A.

89. Cauvin C, Hwang O, Yamamoto M, Van Breeman C (1987) Effects of dihydropyridines on tension and calcium-45 influx in isolated mesenteric resistance vessels from spontaneously hypertensive and normotensive rats. Am J Cardiol 59:116B–122B.

90. Mulvany MJ, Nyborg N (1980): An increased calcium sensitivity of mesenteric resistance vessels in young and adult spontaneously hypertensive rats. Br J Pharmacol 71:585–596.

91. Braunwald E (1982): Mechanism of action of calcium channel blocking agents. N Engl J Med 307:1618–1627.

92. Buhler FR, Hulthen UL, Kiowski W, Muller FB, Bolli P (1982): The place of the calcium antagonist verapamil in antihypertensive therapy. J Cardiovasc Pharmacol 4:s350–s357.

93. Robinson BF, Dobbs RJ, Bayley S (1982): Response of forearm resistance vessels to verapamil and sodium nitroprusside in normotensive and hypertensive men: evidence for a functional abnormality of vascular smooth muscle in primary hypertension. Clin Sci 63:33–42.

94. Rusch NJ, Hermsmeyer RK (1988): Calcium currents are altered on the vascular cell membrane of spontaneously hypertensive rats. Circ Res 63:997–1002.

95. Aoki K, Yamashita K, Tomita N, Tazumi K, Hotta K (1974): ATPase activity and Ca^{++} binding ability of subcellular membrane of arterial smooth muscle in spontaneously hypertensive rats. Jpn Heart J 15:180–181.

96. Webb RC, Bhalla RC (1976): Altered calcium sequestration by subcellular factions of vascular smooth muscle from spontaneously hypertensive rats. J Mol Cell Cardiol 8: 651–661.

97. Kwan C-Y, Belbeck L, Daniel EE (1980): Abnormal biochemistry of vascular smooth muscle plasma membrane isolated from hypertensive rats. Mol Pharmacol 17:137–140.

98. Kwan C-Y, Daniel EE (1987): Arterial muscle membrane abnormalities of hydralazine-treated spontaneously hypertensive rats. Eur J Pharmacol 82:187–190.

99. Chiesi M, Gasser J, Carafoli E (1984): Properties of the Ca-pumping ATPase of sarcoplasmic reticulum from vascular smooth muscle. Biochem Biophys Res Comm 124: 797–806.

100. Wuytack F, Raeymaekers L, Verbist J, De Smedt H, Casteels R (1984): Evidence for the presence in smooth muscle of two types of Ca^{2+}-transport ATPase. Biochem J 224: 445–451.

101. Wuytack F, Casteels R (1980): Demonstration of a (Ca^{2+}-Mg^{2+})-ATPase activity prob-

ably related to Ca^{2+} transport in the microsomal fraction of porcine coronary artery smooth muscle. Biochim Biophys Acta 595:257–263.

102. Carafoli E (1984): Calcium-transporting systems of plasma membranes, with special attention to their regulation. Adv Cyclic Nucl Protein Phosph Res 17:543–549.

103. Matlib MA, Schwartz A, Yamori Y (1985): A Na^+-Ca^{2+} exchange process in isolated sarcolemmal membranes of mesenteric arteries from WKY and SHR rats. Am J Physiol 249:C166–C172.

104. Daniel EE, Kwan C-Y (1981): Control of contraction of vascular muscle—relation to hypertension. Trends Pharmacol Sci 2:207–223.

105. Fleming WW (1980): The electrogenic Na^+,K^+-pump in smooth muscle: physiologic and pharmacologic significance. Ann Rev Pharmacol Toxicol 20:129–149.

106. Overbeck HW, Pamnani MB, Akera T, Brody TM, Haddy FJ (1976): Depressed function of an ouabain-sensitive sodium-potassium pump in blood vessels from renal hypertensive dogs. Circ Res 38 (suppl II):48–52.

107. Webb RC, Bohr DF (1979): Potassium relaxation of vascular smooth muscle from spontaneously hypertensive rats. Blood Vess 16:71–79.

108. Wong SK, Westfall DP, Menear D, Fleming WW (1984): Sodium-potassium pump sites, as assessed by [^{3}H]-ouabain binding, in aorta and caudal artery of normotensive and spontaneously hypertensive rats. Blood Vess 21:211–222.

109. Kahn AM, Shelat H, Allen JC (1986): Na^+-K^+ exhange is present in sarcoleminal vesicles from dog superior mesenteric artery. Am J Physiol 250:H313–H319.

110. Williamson JR (1986): Inositol lipid metabolism and intracellular signaling mechanisms. News Physiol Sci 1:72–76.

111. Little PJ, Cragoe EJ Jr, Bobik A (1986): Na-H exchange is a major pathway for Na influx in rat vascular smooth muscle. Am J Physiol 251:C707–C712.

112. Nabika T, Velletri PA, Beaven MA, Endo J, Lovenberg W (1985): Vasopressin induced calcium increases in smooth muscle cells from spontaneously hypertensive rats. Life Sci 37:579–584.

113. Sugiyama T, Yoshizumi M, Takaku F, et al. (1986): The elevation of the cytoplasmic calcium ions in vascular smooth muscle cells in SHR—measurement of the free calcium ions in single living cells by laser microfluorospectrometry. Biochem Biophys Res Comm 141:340–345.

114. Bukoski RD, DeWan P, McCarron DA (1988): Intracellular Ca^{2+} in cultured aortic myocytes and mesenteric resistance vessels of spontaneously hypertensive and Wistar Kyoto rats. FASEB J 2:A503.

115. Erne P, Resink TJ, Burgisser E, Buhler FR (1985): Platelets and hypertension. J Cardiovasc Pharmacol 7 (suppl 6):S103–S108.

116. Erne P, Bolli P, Burgisser E, Buhler FR (1984): Correlation of platelet calcium with blood pressure: effect of antihypertensive therapy. N Engl J Med 310:1084–1088.

117. Bruschi G, Bruschi ME, Caroppo M, Orlandini G, Spaggiari M, Cavatorta A (1985): Cytoplasmic free [Ca^{2+}] is increased in the platelets of spontaneously hypertensive rats and essential hypertensive patients. Clin Sci 68:179–184.

118. Le Quan Sang KH, Benlian P, Duval C, Montenay-Garestier T, Meyer P, Devynck M-A (1985): Platelet cytosolic-free calcium concentration in primary hypertension. J Hypertens 3:539.

119. Le Quan Sang KH, Devynck M-A (1986): Increased platelet cytosolic free calcium concentration in essential hypertension. J Hypertens 4:567–574.

120. Lechi A, Lechi C, Bonadonna G, et al. (1987): Increased basal and thrombin-induced free calcium in platelets of essential hypertensive patients. Hypertension 9:230–235.

121. Cooper RS, Shamsi N, Katz S (1987): Intracellular calcium and sodium in hypertensive patients. Hypertension 9:224–229.
122. Larsen FL, Katz S, Roufogalis BD, Brooks DE (1981): Physiological shear stresses enhance the Ca^{2+} permeability of human erythrocytes. Nature 294:667–668.
123. Resink TJ, Tkachuk VA, Erne P, Buhler FR (1986): Platelet membrane calmodulin-stimulated calcium-adenosine triphosphatase. Altered activity in essential hypertension. Hypertension 8:159–166.
124. Postnov YV, Orlov SN, Shevchenko A, Adler AM (1977): Altered sodium permeability, calcium binding and Na-K-ATPase activity in the red blood cell membrane in essential hypertension. Pflügers Arch 371:263–369.
125. Postnov YV, Orlov SN, Pokudin NI (1979): Decrease of calcium binding by the red blood cell membrane in spontaneously hypertensive rats and in essential hypertension. Pflügers Arch 379:191–195.
126. Pokudin NI, Orlov SN, Ryashsky GG, Menshikov NY, Tkachuk VA, Postnov YV (1985): Isolation and characteristics of calmodulin from the brain of rats with spontaneous genetic hypertension. Kardiologiia 25:72–77.
127. Vincenzi FF, Morris CD, Kinsel LB, Kenny M, McCarron DA (1986): Decreased in vitro Ca^{2+} ATPase activity in red blood cells of hypertensive subjects. Hypertension 1058–1066.
128. Postnov YV, Orlov SN, Reznikova MB, Rjazhsky GG, Pokudin NI (1984): Calmodulin distribution and Ca^{2+} transport in the erythrocytes of patients with essential hypertension. Clin Sci 66:459–463.
129. Olorunsogo OO, Okudolo BE, Lawal SOA, Falase AO (1985): Erythrocyte membrane Ca^{2+} pumping ATPase of hypertensive humans: reduced stimulation by calmodulin. Biosci Rpt 5:525–531.
130. Lew PD, Favre L, Waldvogel FA, Vallotton MB (1985): Cytosolic free calcium and intracellular calcium stores in neutrophils from hypertensive subjects. Clin Sci 69:227–330.
131. Bruschi G, Bruschi ME, Caroppo M, Orlandini G, Pavarani C, Cavatorta A (1984): Intracellular free $[Ca^{2+}]$ in circulating lymphocytes of spontaneously hypertensive rats. Life Sci 35:535–542.
132. Kowarski S, Cowen LA, Schachter D (1986): Decreased content of integral membrane calcium-binding protein (IMCAL) in tissues of the spontaneously hypertensive rat. Proc Natl Acad Sci (USA) 83:1097–1100.

Nutritional Factors in Hypertension
© *1990 Alan R. Liss, Inc., pages 131–144*

9 | # Dietary Calcium, Sodium, and Hypertension in Blacks and the Elderly

Michael B. Zemel, Ph.D.
James R. Sowers, M.D.

INTRODUCTION

Hypertension occurs with substantially greater frequency among black and elderly Americans than other segments of the U.S. population. When comparable age-sex groups are studied, the incidence of hypertension is two to three times higher in blacks than in whites [79]. Further, the management of hypertension has been reported to be less successful in blacks than whites, although the higher incidence of hypertension is not completely attributable to this factor, as blacks comprise a disproportionately high percentage of both treated and untreated hypertensives [79].

The elderly also exhibit a disproportionately high incidence of hypertension compared to the general U.S. population [88]. Associated with the higher incidence of hypertension in the elderly is an increased risk of congestive heart failure, ischemic heart disease, transient ischemic episodes, and stroke [86]. Thus, while only 20% of the patients in a VA cooperative study were over the age of 60, they accounted for half of the observed cardiovascular morbidity and mortality [98]. This increased cardiovascular risk is associated with the age-related increases in both systolic and diastolic pressure, although systolic hypertension is more closely related to cardiovascular

From the Department of Nutrition and Food Science and Division of Endocrinology and Hypertension (M.B.Z.), and Division of Endocrinology and Hypertension, (J.R.S.) Wayne State University, 160 Old Main Building, 4841 Cass, Detroit, MI 48202, and VA Medical Center, Allen Park, MI 48101 (M.B.Z. and J.R.S.).

risk in the elderly than is diastolic pressure [40,39,80]. This is especially notable because systolic pressure progressively rises with age, while diastolic pressure ceases to increase with age after the age of 60 [81].

The importance of these associations increases as the demographics of our population change. If the elderly are defined, for statistical purposes only, as persons over the age of 65, then the elderly represented only about 4% of the U.S. population in 1900, over 11% (24 million) in 1970, and are projected to comprise approximately 16% of the U.S. population in 2020 [97]. Consequently, the actual number of elderly individuals with hypertension is rising. Results of the 1976–1980 National Health and Nutrition Examination Society (NHANES-II) demonstrate that the prevalence of hypertension increases with age in the United States for both blacks and whites. For all men, the prevalence of hypertension increased by approximately twofold, from 28.4% in the 35–44-year-old group to 60.2% in the 65–74-year-old group. Similarly, women exhibited a threefold increase in the prevalence of hypertension with age, from 19.3% in the 35–44-year-old group to 67.5% in the 65–74-year-old group. Blacks, however, exhibit a more marked age-associated rise in the prevalence of hypertension, with an earlier rise and a higher peak. Thus, the prevalence of hypertension among black females aged 65 to 74 years was 82.9%, versus 67.5% for all females in this age group. Similarly, a higher incidence of hypertension is found in blacks over the age of 75 than in whites over the age of 75, the prevalence rates being 79% and 74% in blacks and whites, respectively.

ROLE OF DIET: POPULATION STUDIES

It is noteworthy that the well-established relationship between age and blood pressure in the United States and other industrialized nations is absent in some primitive, nonindustrialized cultures. Thus, African pygmies, Eskimos, Kalahari bushmen, and tribal South Sea islanders all exhibit little change in blood pressure from early through late adulthood [49,54,55,94]. Although the homogeneity of each of these populations suggests a genetic component to the age-related rise in blood pressure (or lack thereof), other data suggest a strong environmental component. For example, when adults migrate from nonindustrialized areas to urban areas, they develop blood pressure patterns typical of industrialized populations. Differences in diet and physical activity among populations may serve to explain, in part, the absence of age-associated hypertension in some nonindustrialized populations, as these populations generally exhibit higher levels of physical activity and consume less sodium and more potassium and calcium than is typically consumed in Western populations. Similarly, differences in nutrient intake between hypertensives and normotensives, between American blacks and whites, and between elderly and young adults have been reported; these may represent predisposing factors for hypertension.

Although hypertension among blacks and the elderly represents a "salt sensitive" state [52] this salt sensitivity does not appear to be associated with elevated sodium intakes in either group. It has been suggested that, because of the reduced salt taste acuity associated with aging [30], the elderly consume more sodium than young adults. However, Harlan et al. [32,33] reported no association between salt consumption and hypertension in the elderly in the NHANES-I population. Similarly, sodium intake does not appear to be higher in blacks than in whites, and may be slightly lower [46]. Thus, if salt sensitivity among blacks and the elderly is related to diet, nutrients other than sodium must be explored. Evidence is accumulating to indicate that suboptimal intakes of calcium, and possibly potassium, may predispose these populations to salt sensitivity. Harlan et al. [33] reported calcium consumption to be significantly lower in hypertensives than in age-matched normotensives in NHANES-I populations. Similarly, Gualdoni et al. [31] found dietary calcium and potassium to be lower in hypertensive blacks than in either normotensive blacks or whites. It has been suggested that the consistently lower calcium intakes reported by blacks than by whites may be the result of a higher incidence of lactose intolerance in the black population [46].

SALT SENSITIVITY AND SODIUM METABOLISM IN BLACK AND OLDER HYPERTENSIVES

High-sodium diets can increase vascular resistance through a number of mechanisms. Although dietary sodium has been reported to be similar in blacks and Caucasians [46] and in young adults and the elderly [32,33], blacks appear to exhibit a higher sensitivity to dietary sodium. Sodium loading facilitates sympathetic transmission and release of norepinephrine from adrenergic granules [18]. Sodium may also increase vascular smooth muscle tone via effects on transport of vasoactive hormones to receptors and through effects on transmembrane gradients and transport [11,36]. Dietary sodium may increase responses to vasoconstrictor stimuli by increasing cellular sodium and water content and the wall-to-lumen ratio of blood vessels [11,93]. Mark et al. [56] reported that high sodium intakes augmented forearm vasoconstriction in response to cardiopulmonary baroreceptor activation via lower body negative pressure in borderline hypertensives, indicating that sodium loading enhances neurogenic vasoconstriction. This augmentation may result from an effect on central or afferent mechanisms that facilitates neurotransmitter release [18,56]. It should be noted that this neurogenic vasoconstriction was not found in normotensive subjects on high-sodium diets [1,43]. An important central interaction occurs between arterial baroreceptors and cardiopulmonary baroreceptors through vagal afferents [53], and the inhibitory influence of cardiopulmonary receptors is heightened when the inhibitory influence from the arterial baroreceptor is reduced as occurs in borderline hypertension [29,53,92,100]. Thus, exaggerated cardiopulmonary baroreceptor responses to orthostatic stress and to dietary sodium may partially explain the increases in systemic vascular resistance characteristic of hypertension in blacks.

Salt-sensitive states are likely to result, in part, from a reduced ability of the kidneys of blacks and the elderly to appropriately handle a sodium load [50,51]. Luft et al. [51] reported that 94 black subjects exhibited a slower natriuretic response to a sodium load than a group of 74 whites matched for age, weight, body-surface area glomerular filtration rate, and baseline dietary sodium. Impaired natriuretic responses to sodium loads may result from reduced ability to appropriately generate natriuretic subtances, such as dopamine, prostaglandin E_2, and atrial natriuretic peptide. Although norepinephrine levels appear to increase with age [89], a comparable increase in dopamine levels has not been observed; consequently, the senescent kidney may experience a relative deficiency of the natriuretic actions of dopamine relative to norepinephrine levels (i.e., a decrease in the dopamine:norepinephrine ratio). Similarly, recent data from our laboratory indicate that hypertensive blacks exhibit reduced dopamine excretion compared to normotensives in response to both low and high extremes of calcium intake (unpublished data). There is also an age-related reduction in the renal excretion of prostaglandin E_2 [88], a vasodilator with natriuretic properties, and hypertensive blacks appear not to increase prostaglandin excretion in response to dietary sodium.

Intracellular sodium levels are increased in renal arteries, leukocytes, and erythrocytes of people with essential hypertension [20,93,95]. Associated with this phenomenon are several transport abnormalities, including a reduced Km for Na/K ATPase. Consequently, the high incidence of salt sensitivity in the elderly may also be partially related to this phenomenon.

CALCIUM METABOLISM IN SALT SENSITIVITY

Suboptimal calcium intakes [2,25,32,33,61,71] and abnormalities in calcium metabolism [4,17,19,21,28,42,45,48,58,59,60,61,62,63,64,68,69,70, 72,73,75,76,78,84,85,91,101,105,107] may play a role in the genesis and maintenance of hypertension, particularly in the low-renin, salt-sensitive state in humans and in animal models of salt-sensitive hypertension.

Decreased levels of both serum-ionized [84] and total [91] calcium have been reported in patients with essential hypertension compared to normotensives. Similarly, animal models of hypertension, including spontaneously hypertensive rats [66,102] DOCA rats [102] and the New Zealand genetically hypertensive rat [74] have lower serum-ionized and/or total calcium levels than normotensive controls. Further, the calcium bound to the erythrocyte inner membrane surface is reduced in spontaneously hypertensive rats [19,72,76,78] and in human hypertensives [73,76,78]. Calcium ATPase activity is reduced in red blood cells of hypertensives compared to normotensives [99]. The resulting decline in calcium efflux may increase intracellular calcium and, if a comparable effect occurs in vascular smooth muscle, thereby increase vascular tone. However, increasing serum calcium reduced vascular resistance in the New Zealand genetically hypertensive rat and in normotensive rats [70,74] possibly due to a membrane-stabilizing effect of calcium [101].

Resnick et al. [84] reported that hypertensives with low plasma renin activity, characteristic of the salt-sensitive state in both black and the elderly, exhibited a significantly lower level of serum-ionized calcium than either normotensives or high-renin hypertensives. Consistent with this, low-renin hypertensives exhibit significant elevations in circulating parathyroid hormone (PTH) and 1,25-dihydroxyvitamin D levels and a reduction in calcitonin levels compared to normotensives, or to normal and high-renin hypertensives [83].

Elevations in urinary calcium excretion appear to be associated with blood pressure elevation, as low circulating calcium and increased calcium excretion has been observed both in man and in the animal models of hypertension [19,42,66,96,105]. The etiology of this increased urinary calcium loss in hypertension has not been clarified, but may be secondary to alterations in renal tubular handling of sodium. This possibility is supported by several observations. Massrey et al. [57] first noted that an increase in calcium and magnesium excretion occurs in dogs when distal tubular reabsorption of sodium is reduced. Concomitant increases in sodium, calcium, and magnesium excretion were later observed under several different experimental conditions in rats [23,26]. A correlation between net urinary sodium and calcium excretion has also been noted in genetically hypertensive rats [90] and in black subjects with salt-sensitive, low-renin hypertension [105,106]. Recent observations that salt-sensitive, low-renin black hypertensives on low-calcium diets have a significant increase in urinary calcium excretion when their salt intake is increased (Table 1) are consistent with an interrelationship between renal tubular handling of calcium and sodium. Similar relationships between salt intake and increased urinary excretion of calcium has also been observed in the Dahl S model of salt-sensitive hypertension [96]. Thus, in salt-sensitive humans or salt-sensitive animal models of hypertension, the coexistence of increased calcium loss with a suboptimal calcium intake may contribute to a state of calcium deficiency.

Table 1. Urinary Calcium and Sodium Excretion in Hypertensive Black Adults as Affected by Dietary Calcium and Sodium

Mineral (mg/day)	Diet			
	356 mg Ca 1000 mg Na	356 mg Ca 4000 mg Na	956 mg Ca 1000 mg Na	956 mg Ca 4000 mg Na
Calcium	154.9(a)[1] ± 7.7	168.0(b) ± 6.4	153.2(a) ± 7.8	178.9(b) ± 7.7
Sodium	653(a) ± 34	4503(b) ± 304	1027(c) ± 72	5986(d) ± 397

[1]Nonmatching letters in parentheses denote significant (p < 0.05) differences.

Increasing dietary calcium lowers vascular resistance and systemic blood pressure in hypertensive rats [3,4,67,85] while calcium restriction causes vasoconstriction both in spontaneously hypertensive rats and in their normotensive controls [4,41,61]. Further, Belizan et al. [5] reported that 1 gram of elemental calcium per day significantly reduced diastolic blood pressure in men and women in a 22-week placebo-controlled randomized clinical trial; 44% of the 48 hypertensives and 19% of the normotensives experienced a 10 mmHg decrease in systolic pressure. It is noteworthy that consistent changes were not evident until the sixth week of supplementation, and blood pressure declined from 6 weeks until completion of the study. In a longer-term trial, Johnson et al. reported that a 1500 mg/day calcium supplement caused a 13 mmHg reduction in systolic blood pressure in 16 hypertensive postmenopausal women studied over a 4-year period. In contrast, the control group of 18 women given a placebo over the same period of time experienced a 7 mmHg increase. Similarly, in an 8-week randomized double-blind controlled crossover trial, McCarron and Morris found that a 1 g/day calcium supplement significantly reduced systolic pressure in mild to moderate hypertensives, while no significant effect was found in normotensives. However, Belizan et al. found that calcium supplementation of 2 g/day significantly reduced blood pressure in normal pregnant women. Thus, alterations in calcium homeostasis may affect blood pressure regulatory processes and could account for some of the abnormalities in blood pressure regulation seen in salt-sensitive populations, such as black and elderly individuals. This is especially significant in that blacks in the United States consume significantly less calcium than Caucasians [31,46]. This suggests that low levels of calcium intake may be one of the factors responsible for the high incidence of salt sensitivity in this population. Consistent with this concept, we have recently reported that increasing the calcium intake of either normotensive or hypertensive blacks by only 600 mg/day, in the form of yogurt, reverses the sodium-induced elevations in blood pressure found on low-calcium diets [104,106].

Table 2. Effects of Dietary Calcium and Sodium on Supine Systolic and Diastolic Blood Pressure in Salt-sensitive Black Subjects

Measurement	Treatment			
	Low Ca Low Na	Low Ca High Na	High Ca Low Na	High Ca High Na
Systolic pressure (mmHg)	128 ± 4(a)[1]	141 ± 5(b)	128 ± 4(a)	132 ± 5(a)
Diastolic pressure (mmHg)	80 ± 4(a)	84 ± 4(b)	80 ± 3(a)	80 ± 4

[1]Nonmatching letters in parentheses denote significant (p < 0.05) differences.

A relative calcium deficiency would be expected to result in an increase in circulating parathyroid hormone (PTH) and 1,25-dihydroxyvitamin D, for which the signal would presumably be a small, probably transient, decrease in ionized calcium. In accordance with this hypothesis, significant increases in both hormones have been observed in rat models as well as in hypertensive humans [65,66,83,90,91,103,105]. While the role of elevated PTH and 1,25-$(OH)_2$-D in the pathogenesis of salt-sensitive hypertension is not clear, the results of recent studies are instructive. We have recently found that increasing dietary salt at low calcium intakes in low-renin salt-sensitive black hypertensives results in increased serum PTH and urinary cyclic AMP excretion as well as increased blood pressure (Tables 2, and 3). These salt-induced elevations in PTH, urinary cyclic AMP, and blood pressure were abolished by dietary calcium supplementation. These data suggest that the elevations in PTH were due to sodium-induced calciuresis, which may have effected a transient decline in ionized calcium and thereby increased PTH levels. It is especially noteworthy that changes in erythrocyte intracellular calcium paralleled those of PTH (Table 3). Increasing dietary salt at a low level of calcium intake caused a significant increase in intracellular calcium; this elevation in intracellular calcium, as well as the increase in PTH, was abolished by adding calcium to the high-salt diet.

Although these data do not demonstrate a cause-and-effect relationship between the sodium-induced increase in PTH and the observed increase in intracellular calcium, this relationship is predicted as PTH stimulates calcium uptake in several types of cells. If these data from human erythrocytes may be extrapolated to vascular smooth muscle, then these data indicate a potential role for PTH in mediating salt-induced increases in blood pressure, as the PTH may facilitate an increase in vascular smooth muscle cytosolic calcium levels and thereby increase vascular resistance. This concept is supported by data from other tissues, as PTH has been reported to increase calcium uptake in hepatocytes [16], erythrocytes [10], HeLa cells [12], and isolated aorta [87].

Table 3. Serum Mid-molecule Parathyroid Hormone and Erythrocyte Intracellular Calcium in Hypertensive Blacks as Affected by Dietary Calcium and Sodium

Measurement	Diet			
	Low Ca Low Na	Low Ca High Na	High Ca Low Na	High Ca High Na
PTH	0.59(a)[1]	0.65(b)	0.58(a)	0.55(a)
(ng/ml)	±0.08	±0.10	±0.11	±0.13
Intracellular				
calcium	2.16(a)	4.43(b)	2.36(a)	2.20(a)
(μg/ml cells)	±0.27	±1.47	±0.27	±0.30

[1]Nonmatching letters in parentheses denote significant ($p < 0.05$) differences.

Although PTH is recognized to also exert a vasodilatory effect that may be considered paradoxical, this effect may only be manifested at high doses. For example, Schleiffer et al. reported that high levels of parathyroid extract inhibited contraction of isolated aorta in response to phenylephrine, reduced ^{45}Ca influx, and increased ^{45}Ca efflux from isolated rat aorta. In contrast, lower levels of parathyroid extract exerted the opposite effect, increasing ^{45}Ca influx in isolated aorta. Thus, the hypotensive effects of PTH may be realized only under unphysiologically high concentrations that mask the physiological role of PTH as a calcium ionophore and vasoconstrictive agent. Further evidence for such a role of PTH is found in the observation that parathyroidectomy protects Sprague-Dawley rats against mineralocorticoid-induced hypertension, and that cardiovascular reactivity is depressed in thyroparathyroidectomized rats, while autotransplantation of parathyroid glands or PTH administration restores cardiovascular reactivity and the development of hypertension [9]. Further, Gennari et al. [27] reported that the hypertensive effect of acute hypercalcemia is achieved only under intact parathyroid function and is completely abolished by parathyroidectomy. Thus, the hypertensive effects of dietary salt in salt-sensitive individuals may be mediated, in part, by salt-induced increases in PTH and, consequently, in intracellular calcium. It logically follows, then, that the antihypertensive of calcium may result from calcium-induced suppression of PTH and a resultant decrease in intracellular calcium. This may also explain the higher frequency of aging-associated hypertension in blacks compared to Caucasians, as a significantly greater increase in circulating PTH levels with age has been found among blacks.

Recent data suggest an additional mechanism whereby dietary sodium and calcium effect alterations in intracellular calcium, as increasing dietary sodium at a low level of calcium intake caused a significant inhibition of erythrocyte Na/K-ATPase activity and, consequently, a significant increase in intracellular sodium [104]; the increase in intracellular sodium may then cause the observed increase in intracellular calcium by virtue of reduced Na–Ca exchange. Blacks have striking abnormalities of cellular membrane cation transport [35,47,95]. Decreased Na/K ATPase activity [95] may explain the observed increase in intracellular sodium in blacks compared to whites [47,95]. Hilton [35] correlated increases in blood pressure with decreases in Na/K ATPase and increases in intracellular sodium. Since the cellular concentration of calcium is linked, in part, to the transmembrane sodium gradient by a sodium–calcium exchange mechanism, the observed increase in intracellular sodium in blacks may be responsible for the increase in intracellular free calcium found in hypertensives [17,48] and, consequently, for an increase in vascular resistance. Thus, abnormalities in cellular membrane sodium transport may also explain, in part, the marked propensity toward salt sensitivity in the black population. Similar reductions in sodium transport, and presumably increases in intracellular sodium, are associated with aging, as both myocardial and erythrocyte Na/K ATPase activities are decreased with age [23,44]. The sodium-induced decrease in Na/K ATPase and increase in intracellular sodium in blacks are reversed by calcium supplementation [104].

The antihypertensive effects of calcium may also result, in part, from calcium-induced natriuresis and a resultant reduction in intravascular volume. Increasing dietary calcium in salt-sensitive blacks on a moderately high sodium intake caused a significant natriuresis, a reduction in total body water and extracellular water, and an increase in plasma renin activity, indicating reduced intravascular volume [106].

REFERENCES

1. Abboud FM (1974): Effects of sodium, angiotensin and steroids on vascular reactivity in man. Fed Proc 33:143.
2. Ackley S, Barrett-Connor E, Suarez L (1983): Dairy products, calcium and blood pressure. Am J Clin Nutr 38:457–461.
3. Ayachi S (1979): Increased dietary calcium lowers blood pressure in the spontaneously hypertensive rat. Metabolism 28:1234–1238.
4. Belizan JM, Pineda O, Sainz E, Menedez LA, Villar J (1981): Rise of blood pressure in calcium-deprived pregnant rats. Am J Obstet Gynecol 141:153.
5. Belizan JM, Villar J, Pineda O (1983a): Reduction of blood pressure with calcium supplementation in young adults. JAMA 249:1161–1165.
6. Belizan JM, Villar J, Salazar A, Rojas L, Chan D, Bryce GF (1983b): Preliminary evidence of the effect of calcium supplementation on blood pressure in normal pregnant women. Am J Obstet Gynecol 146:175–180.
7. Berthelot A, Gairard A (1980a): Effect of DOCA-saline treatment on calcium metabolism in the rat. Arch Intern De Pharmacodynamic et de Therapi 246:38.
8. Berthelot A, Gairard A (1980b): Parathyroid hormone and deoxycorticosterone acetate induced hypertension in the rat. Clin. Sci. 58:365–371.

9. Berthelot A, Gairard A (1978): Effect of parathyroidectomy on cardiovascular reactivity in rats with mineralocorticoid-induced hypertension. Br J Pharmacol 62:199–205.

10. Bogen E, Massry SG, Levi J, Djaldeti M, Bristol G, Smith J (1982): Effect of parathyroid hormone on osmotic fragility of human erythrocytes. J Clin Invest 69:1017–1025.

11. Bohr DF, Deidel C, Sobieski J (1969): Possible role of sodium-calcium pumps in tension development of vascular smooth muscle. Microvasc Res 1:334.

12. Borle AB (1968): Calcium metabolism in HeLa cells and the effects of parathyroid hormone. J Cell Biol 36:567–582.

13. Brunner HR, Chang P, Wallach R, Sealey JE, Laragh JH (1972): Angiotensin II vascular receptors: Their avidity in relationship to sodium balance, the autonomic nervous system and hypertension. J Clin Invest 51:58–67.

14. Bruschi G, Bruschi ME, Caroppo M, Orlandini G, Spaggiari M, Caotatorta A (1985): Cytoplasmic free (Ca^{2+}) is increased in the platelets of spontaneously hypertensive rats and essential hypertensive patients. Clin Sci 6B:179–184.

15. Canessa M, Adrangna N, Solomon HS, Connolly TM, Tosteson DC (1980): Increased sodium-lithium countertransport in red cells of patients with essential hypertension. N Engl J Med 302:772–776.

16. Chausmer AB, Shermar BS, Wallach S (1982): The effect of parathyroid hormone in hepatic cell transport of calcium. Endocrinology 90:663–672.

17. Cooper RS, Shamsi N, Katz S (1987): Intracellular calcium and sodium in hypertensive patients. Hypertension 9:224–229.

18. DeChamplain J, Krakoff LR, Axelrod J (1968): Relationship between sodium intake and norepinephrine storage during the development of experimental hypertension. Circ Res 23:479.

19. Devynck MA, Pernollet MG, Nunez AM, Meyer P (1981): Analysis of calcium handling in erythrocyte membranes of genetically hypertensive rats. Hypertension 3:397–403.

20. Edmondson RPS, Thomas RD, Hilton PJ, Patrick J, Jones JF (1975): Abnormal leukocyte composition and sodium transport in essential hypertension. Lancet 1:1003–1005.

21. Erne P, Bolli, P, Burgisser E, Buhler FR (1984): Correlation of platelet calcium with blood pressure: Effect of antihypertensive therapy. N Engl J Med 310:1084–1091.

22. Folkow B (1971): Hemodynamic consequences of the adaptive structural changes of the resistance vessels in hypertension. Clin Sci 41:1–12.

23. Gambert SR, Duthie EH (1983): Effect of age on red cell membrane sodium-potassium dependent adenosine triphosphatase (Na^+-K^+ATPase) activity in healthy men. J Gerontol 38:23–28.

24. Garay R, Meyer P (1979): A new test showing abnormal Na and K fluxes in erythrocytes of essential hypertensive patients. Lancet 1:349–353.

25. Garcia-Palmieri MR, Costas R Jr, Cruz-Vidal M, Sorlie PD, Tillotson J, Haylik RJ (1984): Calcium intake and decreased hypertension in Puerto Rico: Puerto Rico Heart Health Program Study. Hypertension 6:322–328.

26. Gairard A, Stoclet JC, Miss C (1973): Evolution du metabolisme calcique durant l'hypertension mineralocorticoide du rat. Cr Soc Biol 167:1977–1982.

27. Gennari C, Nami R, Bianchini C, Aversa AM (1985): Blood pressure effects of acute hypercalcemia in normal subjects and thyroparathyroidectomized patients. Mineral Electrolyte Metab 11:369–373.

28. Grady JR, Dorow J, McCarron DA (1983): Urinary calcium excretion and cAMP response of the spontaneously hypertensive rat. Clin Res 31:330A.

29. Gribbin B, Pickering TG, Sleight P, Peto R (1971): Effect of age and high blood pressure on baroreflex sensitivity in man. Circ Res 29:424–431.

30. Grzegarczyk PB, Jones CW, Mistretta CM (1979): Age related differences in salt taste acuity. J Gerontol 34:834–860.

31. Gualdoni S, Harriman KN, Shugart R, Melville M, Centor R, and Sowers J (1985): Differences in dietary mineral intake and excretion in normotensive and hypertensive blacks and whites. Clin Res 33:(4)850A.

32. Harlan WR, Hull AL, Schmouder RL, Landis JR, Thompson FE, Larkin FA (1984a): Blood pressure and nutrition in adults. Am J Epidemiol 120:17–28.

33. Harlan WR, Hull AL, Schmouder RL, Landis JR, Larkin FA, Thompson FE (1984b): High blood pressure in older Americans: The First National Health and Nutrition Examination Survey. Hypertension 6:802–809.

34. Heistad DD, Abboud FM, Ballard DR (1971): Relationship between plasma sodium concentration and vascular reactivity in man. J Clin Invest 50:2022–2032.

35. Hilton PJ (1986): Cellular sodium transport in essential hypertension. N Engl J Med 314:222–229.

36. Hollander W, Shibata N (1968): Mode of action of sodium on the contractile proteins of the arteries. J Clin Invest 47:47a.

37. Hypertension prevalence and the status of awareness, treatment and control in th United States; (185): Final report of the subcommittee on the definition and prevalence of the 1984 Joint National Committee. Hypertension 7:457–468.

38. Johnson NE, Smith EL, Freudenheim JL (1985): Effects on blood pressure of calcium supplementation of women. Am J Clin Nutr 42:12–17.

39. Kannel WB, Dawber TR, McGee DL (1981): Perspective on systolic hypertension: The Framingham Study. Circulation 61:1179–1182.

40. Kannel WB, Gordon T, Schwartz MJ (1971): Systolic versus diastolic blood pressure and risk of coronary heart disease: The Framingham Study. Am J Cardiol 27:335–346.

41. Karanja N, Metz J, Lee D, Phanouvang T, McCarron DA (1985): Effects of Ca^{2+} and Na^+ on blood pressure, food consumption and weight in the spontaneously hypertensive rat. Kidney Int 27:193.

42. Kesteloot H, Geboers J (1982): Calcium and blood pressure. Lancet 1:813–815.

43. Kirkendall WM, Connor WE, Abbound FM, Rastogi SP, Anderon TA, Fry M (1972): Effect of dietary sodium on the blood pressure of normotensive man. Genest J (ed): International Symposium on Renin-Angiotensin-Aldosterone-Sodium in Hypertension. Springer-Verlag, p 360.

44. Kroening BH, Weintraub M (1980): Age-associated differences in guinea pig myocardial Na^+, K^+ ATPase activity and ouabain inhibition in Mg^{2+} ATPase activity. Pharmacology 21:193–197.

45. Kurtz TW, Morris RC (1985): Dietary CaCl as a determinant of disordered calcium metabolism in the Dahl salt-sensitive rat. Kidney Int 27:194.

46. Langford HG, Langford FPJ, Tyler M (1985): Dietary profile of sodium, potassium and calcium in U.S. blacks. In Hall WD, Saunders E, Shulman NB (eds): "Hypertension in Blacks: Epidemiology, Pathophysiology and Treatment." Chicago: Year Book Medical Publishers, Inc., pp 49–57.

47. Lasker N, Hoop L, Grossman S, Bamforth R, Aviv A (1985): Race and sex differences in erythrocyte Na, K and Na-K adenosine triphosphatase. J Clin Invest 75:1813–1820.

48. Lindner A, Kenny M, Meacham AJ (1986): Effects of a circulating factor in patients with essential hypertension on intracellular free calcium in normal platelets. N Engl J Med 316:509–513.

49. Lovell RRH (1967): Race and blood pressure with special reference to Oceania. In Stamler J, Stamler R, Pullman (eds): "The Epidemiology of Hypertension." New York: Grune and Stratton, pp 122–129.

50. Luft FC, Grim CE, Fineberg N, Weinberger MC (1979): Effects of volume expansion and contraction in normotensive whites, blacks, and subjects of different ages. Circulation 59:643–650.

51. Luft FC, Grim CE, Weinberger MH (1985): Electrolyte and volume homeostasis in blacks. In Hall WP, Saunders E, Shulman WB (eds): "Hypertension in Blacks: Epidemiology, Pathophysiology and Treatment." Chicago: Year Book Medical Publishers, Inc., pp 115–131.

52. Luft FC, Weinberger MH, Fineberg NS, Miller JZ, Grim CE (1987): Effects of age on renal sodium homeostasis and its relevance to sodium sensitivity. Am J Med 82 (suppl 1B):9–15.

53. Mancia G, Shepherd H, Donald D (1976): Interplay among carotid sinus, cardiopulmonary and carotid body reflexes in dogs. Am J Physiol 230:19–24.

54. Mann GV, Roels OA, Price DL, Merril JM (1961): Cardiovascular disease in African Pygmies. J Chronic Dis 15:341–371.

55. Mann GV (1962): The health and nutritional status of Alaskan Eskimos. Am J Clin Nutr 11:31–76.

56. Mark AL, Lawton MD, Fitz AE, Connor WE, Hustad DD (1984): Effects of high and low sodium intake on arterial pressure and forearm vascular resistance in borderline hypertension. Circ Res 36:37.

57. Massry SG, Ciburn JW, Chapman LW, Kleeman CR (1968): The effect of long-term deoxycorticosterone acetate administration on the renal excretion of calcium and magnesium. J Lab Clin Med 71:212–219.

58. McCarron DA (1982a): Blood pressure and calcium balance in the Wistar-Kyoto rat. Life Sci 30:683.

59. McCarron DA (1982b): Low serum concentrations of ionized calcium in patients with hypertension. N Engl J Med 307:226–228.

60. McCarron DA (1982c): Calcium, magnesium, phosphorus balance in human and experimental hypertension. Hypertension 4 (suppl III):27.

61. McCarron DA, Lucas PA, Lacour B, Shneidman RJ, Drucke T (1985): Blood pressure development of the spontaneously hypertensive rat following concurrent manipulation of dietary Ca^{2+} and Na^+: Relation to intestinal Ca^{2+} fluxes. J Clin Invest 76:1147–1154.

62. McCarron DA, Morris CD (1985a): Blood pressure response to oral calcium in persons with mild to moderate hypertension. Ann. Int. Med. 103:825–831.

63. McCarron DA, Morris CD, Cole C (1983): Dietary calcium in human hypertension. Science 217:267–269.

64. McCarron DA, Morris CD, Staton JL (1984b): Blood pressure and nutrients in the United States. Science 224:1392–1398.

65. McCarron DA, Pinyree PA, Rubin RJ, Gaucher SM, Molitch M, Krutzik S (1980): Enhanced parathyroid function in essential hypertension: A homeostatic response to a urinary calcium leak. Hypertension 2:162–168.

66. McCarron DA, Yung NN, Ugoretz BA, Krutzik S (1981): Disturbances of calcium metabolism in the spontaneously hypertensive rat. Hypertension 3:I-162–167.

67. McCarron DA, Wegener LL (1985b): Pressor response to angiotensin II in the SHR: Modification by dietary calcium and sodium. Clin Res 33:364A.

68. Morris CD, Vincenzi F, McCarron DA (1985): Ca^{2+}, ATPase activity in human hypertension. Kidney Int 27:197.

69. Morris RC, Kurtz TW (1985): Dietary chloride as a determinant of disordered calcium metabolism in deoxycorticosteroid hypertension. Kidney Int 27:196.

70. Mulvany MJ, Korsgaard N, Nyborg N (1981): Evidence that the increased calcium

sensitivity of resistance vessels in spontaneously hypertensive rats is an intrinsic defect of the vascular smooth muscle. Clin Exp Hypertens (A)3:749–761.

71. Nichaman M, Shekelle R, Paul O (1984): Diet, alcohol, and blood pressure in the Western Electric Study. Am J Epidemiol 120:469–470.

72. Orlov SN, Pokudin NI, Postnov YV (1983): Calmodulin-dependent Ca-transport in erythrocytes of spontaneously hypertensive rats. Pflügers Arch 397:54–56.

73. Orlov SN, Postnov YV (1982): Ca^{2+} binding and membrane fluidity in essential and renal hypertension. Clin Sci 63:281–284.

74. Overbeck HW (1984): Attenuated arteriolar dilator responses to calcium in genetically hypertensive rats. Hypertension 6:647–653.

75. Postnov YV, Orlov SN, Pokudin NI (1980): Alteration of intracellular calcium distribution in adipose tissue of human patients with essential hypertension. Pflügers Arch 388:89–91.

76. Postnov YV, Orlov SN, Pokudin NI (1979): Decrease of calcium binding by the red blood cell membrane in spontaneously hypertensive rats and in essential hypertension. Pflügers Arch 379:191–195.

77. Postnov YV, Orlov SN, Reznikova MB, Rjazhsky GG, Pokudin NI (1984): Calmodulin distribution of Ca^{2+} transport in the erythrocytes of patients with essential hypertension. Clin Sci 66:459–465.

78. Postnov YV, Orlov SN, Shevchenko A, Alder AM (1977): Altered sodium permeability, calcium binding and Na-K-ATPase activity in the red blood cell membrane in essential hypertension. Pflügers Arch 371:263–269.

79. Prineas RJ and Gillum R (1985): U.S. epidemiology of hypertension in blacks. In Hall WD, Saunders E, Shulman NB (eds): "Hypertension in Blacks: Epidemiology, Pathophysiology and Treatment." Chicago: Year Book Medical Publishers, Inc., pp 17–36.

80. Rabbin SW, Motherson RAL, Tate RB (1978): Predicting risk of ischemic heart disease and cerebrovascular disease from systolic and diastolic pressure. Ann Intern Med 88: 342–345.

81. Reed G, Anderson RJ (1982): Hypertension in the elderly. Clin Ther 5:1–38.

82. Reed D, McGee D, Yano K, Hankin J (1984): Diet, blood pressure and multicollinearity. Hypertension 7:405–410.

83. Resnick LM (1987): Uniformity and diversity of calcium metabolism in hypertension. A conceptual framework. Am J Med 82 (suppl 1B):16–26.

84. Resnick LM, Laragh JH, Sealey JE, Alderman MH (1983): Divalent cations in essential hypertension: Relations between serum ionized calcium, magnesium and plasma renin activity. N Engl J Med 309:888–891.

85. Robinson BF (1984): Altered calcium handling as a cause of primary hypertension. J Hypertension 2:453–457.

86. Rudin AM, Black HR (1981): Hypertension in the elderly: the time has come to treat. Am Geriatr Soc 29:193–200.

87. Schleiffer R, Berthelot A, Gairard (1979): Effects of parathyroid extract on blood pressure and arterial contraction of ^{45}Ca exchange in isolated aorta in the rat. Blood Vessels 16:220–221.

88. Sowers JR (1987): Hypertension in the elderly. Am J Med 82 (suppl 1B):1–8.

89. Sowers JR, Rubenstein LZ, Stern N (1983): Plasma norepinephrine responses to posture and isometric exercise increase with age in the absence of obesity. J Gerontol 38: 315–317.

90. Stern N, Lee D, Silis V, Beck F, Deftos L, Monolagas S, Sowers JR (1984): The effects of high calcium intake on blood pressure and calcium metabolism in the young spontaneously hypertensive rat. Hypertension 6:639–646.

91. Strazzulo P, Nunziata V, Cirillo M, Giannattasio R, Mancini M (1983): Abnormalities of calcium metabolism in essential hypertension. Clin Sci 65:137–141.
92. Takeshita A, Tanaka S, Nakmura M (1979): Reduced baroreceptor sensitivity in borderline hypertension. Circulation 59:632–636.
93. Tobian L Jr, Binion JT (1952): Tissue cations and water in arterial hypertension. Circulation 5:745.
94. Truswell AS, Hansen JDL (1976): Medical research among the Kung. In Lee RB, DeVore I (eds): "Kalahari Hunter-Gatherers: Harvard University Press.
95. Tuck ML, Gross C, Maxwell MH, Brickman AS, Krasnoshtein G, Mayes D (1984): Erythrocyte Na, K cotransport and Na, K pump in black and Caucasian hypertension patients. Hypertension 6:536–544.
96. Ummemura S, Smyths DD, Nicar M, Rapp JP, Pettinger WA (1986): Altered calcium homeostasis in Dahl hypertensive rats: Physiological and biochemical studies. J Hypertension 4:19–26.
97. U.S. Bureau of the Census (1978): Current population reports. Series P-25.
98. Veterans Administration (1972): Veterans Administration Cooperative Study Group on Antihypertensive Agents: Effects of treatment on morbidity in hypertension. III. Influence of age, diastolic pressure, and prior cardiovascular diseases, further analysis of side effects. Circulation 45:999–1004.
99. Vincenzi FF, Morris CD, Kinsel LB, Kenny M, McCarron DA (1986): Decreased calcium pump adenosine triphosphatase in red blood cells of hypertensive subjects. Hypertension 8:1058–1066.
100. Volpe M, Tremarco B, Ricciardelli B (1982): The autonomic nervous tone abnormalities in the genesis of the impaired baroreflex responsiveness in borderline hypertensive subjects. Clin Sci 62:581–588.
101. Webb RC, Bohr DF (1978): Mechanism of membrane stabilization by calcium in vascular smooth muscles. Am J Physiol 235:C227–232.
102. Wright GL, Rankin GO (1982): Concentrations of ionic and total calcium in plasma of four models of hypertension. Am J Physiol 243:(suppl):H365–370.
103. Zemel MB, Allison T, Gualdoni S, Zemel P, Sowers J (1986a): Age related changes in serum total and ionized calcium in black and Caucasian males. Clin Res 34:489A.
104. Zemel MB, Kraniak J, Standley P, Gualdoni SM, Komanicky P, Sowers JR (1987): Effects of dietary sodium and calcium on cellular calcium, magnesium, sodium and potassium metabolism in hypertensive blacks. Clin Res 35:452A.
105. Zemel MB, Gualdoni SM, Walsh MF, Komanicky P, Standley P, Johnson D, Fitter W, Sowers JR (1986b): Effects of sodium and calcium on calcium metabolism and blood pressure regulation in hypertensive black adults. J Hypertension 4 (suppl 5):S364–S366.
106. Zemel MB, Gualdoni SM, Sowers JR (1986c): Sodium excretion and plasma renin activity in normotensive and hypertensive black adults as affected by dietary calcium and sodium. J Hypertension 4(suppl 6):5343–5345.
107. Zidek W, Vetter H, Dorst KG, Zumkley H, Losse H (1982): Intracellular Na^+ and Ca^{2+} activities in essential hypertension. Clin Sci 63:413–418.

Nutritional Factors in Hypertension
© 1990 Alan R. Liss, Inc., pages 145–154

| 10 | Cellular Mechanisms Related to the Antihypertensive Effect of Calcium: Vascular Smooth Muscle As an Example |

Frank F. Vincenzi, Ph.D.

INTRODUCTION

It is well established that serum-ionized calcium (I will here refer to Ca as the free ion, Ca^{2+}, unless otherwise specified) is regulated at approximately 10^{-3} M in a wide variety of mammalian organisms. Likewise, it is quite clear that intracellular Ca is maintained at 10^{-7} M or less in "resting" cells [15,21,29]. This condition appears to be rather universal among living cells. Thus, there is a gradient across the plasma membrane of 10,000 to 1 or more. Because intracellular Ca is very low, it is possible for cells to allow the entry of small amounts of Ca and use the resultant transient increases as a signaling mechanism. Cells have developed a variety of mechanisms for increasing cytosolic Ca. Several mechanisms also exist to remove Ca from the cytosol. One possible basis of the increased peripheral resistance characteristic of much essential hypertension is an alteration in the balance of the processes that maintain low intracellular Ca in vascular smooth muscle.

CALCIUM ENTRY

Channels in the plasma membrane appear to be responsible for the majority of influx of Ca into most cells [2]. Ca channels are generally considered to be receptor-operated channels (ROCs) or voltage-operated channels (VOCs). Receptors on the surface of the plasma membrane couple to the

From the Department of Pharmacology, SJ-30, University of Washington, Seattle WA 98195.

former type of Ca channel. A wide variety of agonist molecules, including acetylcholine, histamine, and serotonin, converge through their respective receptors on what appears to be a common population of receptor-operated channels. These ROCs open in response to occupation of a receptor by the agonist molecule. The resultant influx of Ca can be sufficient to stimulate muscle contraction, hormone release, or whatever is an appropriate response of the effector cell. Much like Na channels, VOCs are controlled by membrane voltage. They are opened transiently by depolarization. They also exhibit inactivation and other features typical of voltage-operated channels [27]. A complex interplay of agonist and antagonist effect on ROCs and indirectly via alterations in membrane voltage accounts for much of the effects of chemicals on smooth muscle.

BLOCKADE OF CALCIUM ENTRY

A number of agents have been discovered that interfere with the activity of Ca channels. The widespread importance of Ca in cellular function undoubtedly accounts for the wide therapeutic usefulness of Ca channel blockers in a variety of conditions.

Effective Ca channel blockers differ from one another structurally, although functionally they have similar but not identical properties. Verapamil, diltiazem, and nifedipine, for example, have in common that they are amphipathic molecules. They tend to bind in the membrane and interfere with the conducting properties of both VOCs and ROCs. Thus, they can effectively reduce the influx of Ca into cells under a variety of circumstances.

Therefore, if one is in the difficult position, for example, of trying to prevent spasm of coronary muscle as caused by some generally unknown circulating chemical which activates ROCs, it is nearly hopeless to try to block all of the surface receptors upon which the unknown agent might potentially be acting. But an agent that blocks the common mechanism through which most of the surface active agents work to increase intracellular Ca can be appropriate and effective in such a case. Such effectiveness accounts for the immense popularity of the Ca channel blockers in the treatment of angina pectoris, thought in many cases to be mediated by spasm of coronary arteries.

Ca channel blockers have in common that they limit the ratio of intracellular Ca compared to extracellular Ca. Admittedly, such agents have different effects on different cell types, but the common mechanism appears to be useful in a wide variety of conditions such as angina, cardiac arrhythmias, and hypertension. Presumably, in hypertension Ca channel blockers reduce the entry of Ca into vascular smooth muscle and thereby reduce peripheral vascular resistance.

INTRACELLULAR CALCIUM RELEASE

In some cells, especially skeletal muscle, there is a good deal of internal release of Ca. Both electrically and chemically [10] mediated release of Ca from internal stores have been demonstrated. Ca released from internal stores augments the signal produced by Ca influx and can be the major source of "trigger" Ca for physiological responses in some cells (e.g., skeletal muscle).

A special case of chemically induced release of intracellular Ca has recently come to light. Some cell surface agonists stimulate the production of inositol triphosphate (IP3) at the inner surface of the plasma membrane. It is now recognized that IP3 releases intracellular stored Ca via interaction with specific receptors, presumably on the surface of the endoplasmic reticulum [3]. Whether the metabolism of IP3 is altered in hypertension is unknown. Abnormally large production and/or decreased destruction of IP3 could conceivably underlie an abnormally elevated intracellular Ca, or at least the magnitude of the "pulses" of Ca released by certain agonists that promote IP3 production.

CALCIUM EXTRUSION

The amount of Ca available for signaling in a cell is a balance of the Ca that is internally released and that which enters across the plasma membrane minus that which is ejected and/or stored. It is very important for any signal in biology to be terminated, or else it may become a pathological signal. This is also true for intracellular Ca signals. In order that the intracellular Ca signal be only transient in the face of a tremendous inward gradient, cells have developed several ways to achieve and maintain low cytosolic Ca. These mechanisms include a plasma membrane Ca pump that extrudes Ca [24], a plasma membrane Na/Ca exchanger that extrudes Ca under some conditions [5], an endoplasmic reticulum membrane Ca pump [17], and mitochondrial Ca uptake [7]. The latter two processes serve only to decrease cytosolic free Ca and store Ca in the cell without removing it. The former two processes, as variably expressed and active in different cells and different physiological and/or pathological conditions, presumably account for long-term balance of the Ca content of cells. Thus, considerations of chronic imbalance of cellular distribution of Ca must include concern with plasma membrane influx and efflux. Evidence for Na/Ca exchange in smooth muscle is equivocal. The exchanger clearly operates to remove Ca from heart muscle [8], but in cells with a lower average membrane potential the exchanger may serve as a "balanced exchanger" or even serve as a Ca influx pathway [25]. Thus, I will emphasize the Ca pump in this discussion.

The plasma membrane Ca pump, like the Na, K pump, is linked to the activity of a membrane-bound adenosine triphosphatase (ATPase) [24]. The ATPase is activated by Ca at the inner surface of the plasma membrane with a threshold of approximately 10^{-7} M [31]. Its high affinity is necessary in order to maintain the extremely low level of Ca in the cell. The Ca pump is probably present in all cells, whether they move large amounts of Ca or not. The Ca pump and its ATPase is activated by calmodulin (CaM) [16] and is inhibited by anti-CaM drugs such as trifluoperazine [14,20]. Although it is an ATPase, like the Na, K pump ATPase, it is a separate and distinct pump. It is not inhibited by ouabain, as is the Na, K pump. We would know more about the Ca pump if we had a potent and specific inhibitor for it.

CALCIUM-MEDIATED MUSCLE CONTRACTION

If an appropriate transient increase in cytosolic Ca occurs in a muscle cell, then interaction between myosin and actin is activated and contraction occurs. But the mechanism is different in striated as compared to smooth muscle. If one isolates myosin and actin from striated (heart or skeletal) muscle, then they interact automatically and split ATP. This in vitro splitting of ATP is the test-tube equivalent of muscle contraction. In other words, actin and myosin of striated muscle tend to "contract," given a source of ATP. On the other hand, in the presence of the regulatory proteins (the tropomyosin complex containing troponin I, troponin T, and troponin C) from the muscle cell, there is an inhibition of the interaction between actin and myosin. If Ca is then added, actin and myosin are activated. In other words, in striated muscle, the regulatory proteins inhibit the interaction of actin and myosin, and a transient pulse of Ca—ionically and transiently—disinhibits the actin and myosin and allows them to interact [9].

If, on the other hand, actin and myosin are isolated from smooth muscle and incubated in the presence of ATP, little or no ATP splitting occurs [9]. But if the regulatory proteins of smooth muscle (CaM, and myosin light chain kinase) are added, then ATP is split (i.e., the actin and myosin "contract"). Smooth muscle appears to be turned on "covalently." Increased Ca in the cytosol of smooth muscle promotes an interaction with the ubiquitous and universal intracellular Ca receptor protein, CaM. When CaM is complexed with Ca, it in turn forms a complex with myosin light chain kinase. This activates the enzymatic activity of myosin light chain kinase [26]. Myosin light chain kinase is an enzyme that promotes the phosphorylation of the "light chain" of myosin. When the light chain of smooth muscle myosin is phosphorylated, contraction occurs. So in smooth muscle as compared to striated muscle, the contraction is covalently activated [1]. Phosphorylation is thus the "on switch" for muscle contraction and the "switch-off" occurs via myosin phosphatase, the regulation of which is poorly understood at this time [26]. Thus, the fundamental issue in smooth muscle contraction is to get an increase in cytosolic Ca, which forms the complex with CaM, which activates myosin light chain kinase, which phosphorylates the light chains of myosin, which leads to contraction.

It must be emphasized that this presentation is a somewhat simplified approach. For example, producing an increase in cytosolic Ca is not a trivial matter. Even within vascular smooth muscle there are significant differences in the effects of Ca and Ca entry blockers from one vascular bed to another [28]. Part of the differential sensitivity to agents that block the entry of Ca may be related to different dependencies on intracellular release of Ca in different vascular smooth muscle [4]. An alternate view of the activation of smooth muscle contraction relates to the activity of protein kinase C [19].

If one exposes smooth muscle to an agonist or potassium to depolarize the muscle, one typically sees an early phasic contraction and then a maintained tone. Based on the work from a variety of laboratories, it is known that the early phasic contraction is based on the release of Ca from modest internal stores of Ca in smooth muscle [12]. By contrast, in order to maintain tone in smooth muscle, plasma membrane influx must occur. This is flux mediated by Ca channels. Ca continues to enter under conditions that maintain smooth muscle tone. Presumably, a kind of new steady state exists in stimulated smooth muscle with increased rates of both influx and efflux (mediated mainly via the plasma membrane Ca pump). It is possible that slight changes in the balance of influx to efflux are responsible for the elevated intracellular Ca in hypertension. This could arise from too many active Ca channels— channels that remain open over too great a range of voltages, or channels that remain open abnormally long in response to a given stimulus. Alternatively, decreased Ca efflux could result in a greater steady state of intracellular Ca. Naturally, other variations are possible. In any event, such an altered balance of intracellular to extracellular Ca is postulated to account for a significant fraction of essential hypertension. Elucidation of the mechanism(s) responsible may lead to more rational therapy than now exists.

ELEVATED INTRACELLULAR CALCIUM IN HYPERTENSION?

It is generally, but not universally [13], agreed that increased peripheral vascular resistance is a cardinal feature of most cases of established hypertension. Increased intracellular Ca, particularly in vascular smooth muscle

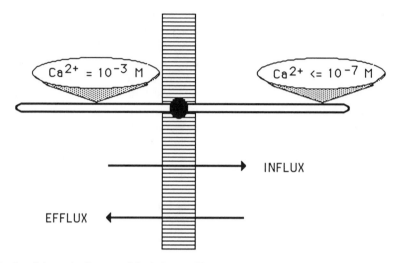

Fig. 1. Schematic diagram of the balance of intracellular and extracellular Ca. Intracellular Ca is maintained at or below 10^{-7} M in the face of 10^{-3} M extracellular Ca. Over relatively long periods of time the amount of Ca entering the cell must be balanced by the amount of Ca leaving the cell. A slight modification of this balance in favor of elevated intracellular Ca may exist in vascular smooth muscle in hypertension.

may thus be fundamental to a significant fraction of what is presently called essential hypertension. This is obviously a simple hypothesis, but it needs to be eliminated if more complex ideas are to be seriously considered.

In order to consider this idea, one should consider the balance of Ca influx and efflux. This balance is depicted schematically in Figure 1. The figure is intended to emphasize that long-term regulation of the amount of free Ca in cells is dependent upon a balance of the influx and efflux of Ca. Changes in either one or both of these fluxes could result in a change in the level of free intracellular Ca. If it is assumed that processes responsible for maintaining extracellular Ca (such as parathyroid hormone, vitamin D, and calcitonin) are not affected (in, for example, hypertension), then an imbalance in plasma membrane fluxes of Ca would result in altered intracellular Ca.

If intracellular Ca were elevated slightly and chronically in vascular smooth muscle, could such an abnormality be fundamental in hypertension? Data are available that show elevated intracellular Ca in platelets of patients with hypertension [11]. Furthermore, an excellent correlation was found between the level of intracellular Ca and the blood pressure of the patients. Of course, such data do not demonstrate but are compatible with a causal link between the two variables.

Thus, it is a hypothesis of some attractiveness that, in at least some kinds of essential hypertension, a defect exists in the regulation of intracellular Ca as compared to extracellular Ca. An abnormally elevated intracellular Ca could (by mechanisms to be discussed below) subserve increased vascular tone and peripheral vascular resistance, commonly recognized as an underlying cardiovascular abnormality in established hypertension. Such a hypothesized abnormally high intracellular Ca might occur even in the face of a normal (or even decreased) extracellular Ca if the balance between intracellular and extracellular Ca were disturbed. Most investigators have found that extracellular Ca is normal or somewhat low in hypertensives [18,22]. It must be admitted that mechanisms by which the balance of intracellular to extracellular Ca may be disturbed in hypertension are unknown, as are mechanism(s) by which calcium supplementation of the diets lowers blood pressure in a significant fraction of subjects with mild to moderate hypertension.

A DEFICIT IN THE CALCIUM PUMP IN HYPERTENSION?

As a first approach to the question of whether a generalized defect in the plasma membrane Ca pump ATPase exists in hypertension, we measured its activity in human RBC membranes. For this assay we examined the ATPase activities (defined operationally by various inclusions in the assay medium) of saponin lysates of washed RBCs. Blood samples were obtained from normotensives and hypertensives who were part of a study of the effects of dietary Ca supplementation on blood pressure. No effect of dietary Ca was noted on any ATPase activity. On the other hand, the basal Ca pump ATPase activity (that measured in the presence of 10^{-4} M TFP) was significantly lower in hypertensive than in normotensive RBC lysates [30]. Although each ATPase had somewhat less activity in hypertensive than normotensive lysates, no other ATPase activity, including the maximal, CaM-activated Ca pump ATPase, differed significantly. The significance of these observations remains to be determined, but may support the notion of a moderate impairment of the plasma membrane Ca pump in human hypertension.

MECHANISM OF DIETARY CALCIUM ON BLOOD PRESSURE?

It appears that in approximately 40% of humans with mild to moderate hypertension, Ca supplementation of the diet lowers mean arterial blood pressure by 10 mmHg or more [18]. The mechanism(s) by which this occurs are not understood.

In fact, how can one make sense out of the observation that Ca channel blockers are useful in the treatment of hypertension and yet also that one can successfully treat hypertensives with dietary Ca? How can it be that Ca entry blockers, on the one hand, and Ca on the other hand, can each (separately or maybe even together) be useful in the treatment of hypertension? I would like to suggest that the evidence available to date is compatible with several possible interpretations. One interpretation is that extracellular Ca itself is a "physiological" Ca entry blocker. Some investigators have found that serum-ionized Ca is decreased in some human hypertension, and it has been shown in several laboratories that it is also decreased in hypertension in animals. And dietary supplementation can lower blood pressure in some hypertensives [18].

Based on work in a number of laboratories, Ca at the outer surface of the plasma membrane seems to "stabilize" the membrane and seems to reduce the effectiveness of Ca channels. Some investigators suggest that Ca that comes through the channel signals the channel to inactivate. In any event, slight increases in extracellular Ca can have the effect of reducing the effectiveness of both receptor-operated and voltage-operated Ca channels. So Ca at the external surface of the membrane may in fact be a kind of Ca entry blocker. It is suggested that increased Ca in the diet results in an alteration of the regulation of intracellular vs. extracellular Ca. How this may occur may seem paradoxical. One possibility is that extracellular Ca acts as what would a few years ago have been termed a "stabilizer" of the smooth muscle membrane [6]. Now it would be fashionable to suggest that Ca may be a rather physiological Ca channel blocker. That is, Ca on the outer surface of the PM may reduce the effectiveness of Ca channels through a mechanism yet to be determined.

Another interpretation that is consistent with the data is that the sensitivity to intracellular Ca is increased in hypertension compared to normal. Other obvious possibilities include dietary Ca-induced changes in the relative amounts or effectiveness of unknown circulating "factors" that may promote hypertension [23]. In any event, it is apparent that Ca supplementation of the diet can result in decreased blood pressure in a significant subpopulation of hypertensives. The mechanism(s) by which this occurs remains to be elucidated.

SUMMARY

It is suggested that in at least some forms of hypertension a subtle abnormality exists such that the normal relationship between extracellular free Ca and intracellular free Ca is shifted toward increased intracellular free Ca. Several mechanisms by which this might occur are considered. None is proven. The possible mechanism(s) by which calcium supplementation of the diet lowers blood pressure in hypertension remains to be determined.

NOTE ADDED IN PROOF

Since the writing of this chapter, we obtained data that do not support the existence of a generalized defect in the plasma membrane Ca pump associated with human hypertension [Vincenzi FF, Di Julio D, Morris DD, McCarron DA (1988): Measurements on the activity of the plasma membrane Ca pump ATPase in human hypertension. In Bronner F, Peterlik M (eds): "Cellular Calcium and Phosphate Transport in Health and Disease." New York: Alan R. Liss, pp 379–383]. Therefore, my laboratory is pursuing the idea of circulating factors that may inhibit the Ca pump.

REFERENCES

1. Adelstein RS, deLanerolle P, Sellers JR, Pato MD, Conti MA (1982): The regulation of myosin light chain kinase of Ca^{++} and calmodulin *in vitro* and *in vivo*. In Kakiuchi S, Hidaka H, Means AR (eds): "Calmodulin and Intracellular Ca^{++} Receptors." New York: Plenum Press, pp 313–331.
2. Almers W, McCleskey EW, Palade PT (1985): Calcium channels in vertebrate skeletal muscle. In Rubin RP, Weiss GB, Putney JW (eds): "Calcium in Biological Systems." New York: Plenum Press, pp 321–330.
3. Berridge MJ (1985): Calcium-mobilizing receptors membrane phosphoinositides and signal transduction. In Rubin RP, Weiss GB, Putney JW (eds): "Calcium in Biological Systems." New York: Plenum Press, pp 37–44.
4. Bevan JA, McCalden TA, Rapoport RM (1981): Differential effects of calcium entry blockers on vascular smooth muscle. In Weiss GB (ed): "New Perspectives on Calcium Antagonists." Bethesda: American Physiological Society, pp 123–129.
5. Blaustein MP, Nelson MT (1982): Sodium-calcium exchange: Its role in the regulation of cell calcium. In Carafoli E (ed): New York: Academic Press, pp 217–236.
6. Bohr DF (1963): Vascular smooth muscle: dual effect of calcium. Science 139:597–599.
7. Bygrave FL, Reinhart PH, Taylor WM (1985): Mitochondrial calcium fluxes and their role in the regulation of intracellular calcium. In Marme D (ed): "Calcium and Cell Physiology." New York: Springer-Verlag, pp 94–104.
8. Carafoli E (1985): The homeostasis of calcium in heart cells. J Mol Cell Cardiol 17: 203–212.
9. Ebashi S, Nakamura S, Nakasoni H, Kohama K, Nonomura Y (1982): Differences and similarities of contractile mechanism in muscle. In Godfraind T, Albertini A, Paoletti R (eds): "Calcium Modulators." New York: Elsevier Biomedical Press, pp 39–49.
10. Endo M, Kitazawa T (1985): Calcium ions and contraction of smooth muscle by alpha-adrenergic stimulation. In Godfraind T, Vanhoutte PM, Govoni S, Paoletti R (eds): "Calcium Entry Blockers and Tissue Protection." New York: Raven Press, pp 81–89.
11. Erne P, Burgisser E, Bolli P, Ji B, Buhler FR (1984): Free calcium concentration in platelets closely relates to blood pressure in normal and essentially hypertensive subjects. Hypertension 6 (suppl 1):166–169.
12. Fleckenstein-Gruen (1982): Control of coronary spasms by calcium antagonists. In Godfraind T, Albertini A, Paoletti R (eds): "Calcium Modulators." New York: Elsevier Biomedical Press, pp 141–154.
13. Guyton AC (1980): "Arterial Pressure and Hypertension." Philadelphia: W.B. Saunders Company, pp 1–9.

14. Hinds TR, Raess BU, Vincenzi FF (1981): Plasma membrane Ca^{2+} transport: antagonism by several potential inhibitors. J Membrane Biol 58:57–65.

15. Itano T, Penniston JT (1985): Ca^{2+}-pumping ATPase of plasma membranes. In Hidaka H, Hartshorne DJ (eds): "Calmodulin Antagonists and Cellular Physiology." New York: Academic Press, pp 335–345.

16. Larsen FF, Vincenzi FF (1979): Ca^{2+} transport across the plasma membrane: Stimulation by calmodulin. Science 204:306–309.

17. Martonosi AN (1975): The mechanism of calcium transport in sarcoplasmic reticulum. In Carafoli E, Clementi F, Drabikowski W Margreth A (eds): "Calcium Transport in Contraction and Secretion." New York: American Elsevier Publishing Company, pp 313–327.

18. McCarron DA (1985): Calcium in the pathogenesis and therapy of human hypertension. Am J Med 78 (suppl 2B):27–34.

19. Park S, Rasmussen H (1985): Activation of tracheal smooth muscle contraction: Synergism between Ca^{2+} and activators of protein kinase C. Proc Natl Acad Sci USA 82: 8835–8839.

20. Raess BU, Vincenzi FF (1980): Calmodulin activation of red blood cell (Ca^{2+} + Mg^{2+})-ATPase and its antagonism by phenothiazines. Molec Pharmacol 18:253–258.

21. Rega AF (1986): The cellular calcium. In Rega AF, Garrahan PJ (eds): "The Ca^{2+} Pump of Plasma Membranes." Boca Raton: CRC Press, pp 1–11.

22. Resnick L (1986): Calcium metabolism, renin activity, and the antihypertensive effects of calcium channel blockade. Am J Med 81 (suppl 6A):6–14.

23. Sagnella GA, Jones JC, Shore AC, Markandu ND, MacGregor GA (1986): Evidence for increased levels of a circulating ouabain-like factor in essential hypertension. Hypertension 8:433–437.

24. Schatzmann HJ, Vincenzi FF (1969): Calcium movements across the membrane of human red cells. J Physiol 201:369–395.

25. Snowdowne KW, Borle AB (1985): Effects of low extracellular sodium on cytosolic ionized calcium. J Biol Chem 260:14998–15007.

26. Stull JT, Blumenthal DK, Botterman BR, Klug GA, Manning DR, Silver PJ (1982): The regulation of myosin light chain kinase by Ca^{++} and calmodulin *in vitro* and *in vivo*. In Kakiuchi S, Hidaka H, Means AR (eds): "Calmodulin and Intracellular Ca^{++} Receptors." New York: Plenum Press, pp 219–238.

27. Trautwein W, Pelzer (1985): Voltage-dependent gating of single calcium channels in the cardiac cell membrane and its modulation by drugs. In Marme D (ed): "Calcium and Cell Physiology." New York: Springer-Verlag, pp 53–93.

28. Vanhoutte PM (1981): Differential effects of calcium entry blockers on vascular smooth muscle. In Weiss GB (ed): "New Perspectives on Calcium Antagonists." Bethesda: American Physiological Society, pp 109–121.

29. Vincenzi FF, Hinds TR (1980): Calmodulin and plasma membrane calcium transport. In Cheung WY (ed): "Calcium and Cell Function, Vol. 1." New York: Academic Press, pp 127–165.

30. Vincenzi FF, Morris CD, Kinsel LB, Kenny M, McCarron DA (1986): Decreased *in vitro* Ca^{2+} pump ATPase activity in red blood cells of hypertensive subjects. Hypertension 8:1058–1066.

31. Vincenzi FF, Schatzmann (1967): Some properties of Ca-activated ATPase in human red cells. Helv Physiol Pharmacol Acta 25:CR233–CR234.

Nutritional Factors in Hypertension
© *1990 Alan R. Liss, Inc., pages 155–173*

| 11 | # Mechanisms of Action of Calcium Absorption Factors That Influence Bioavailability |

Tilman B. Drüeke, M.D.

INTRODUCTION

The bioavailability of calcium is regulated by three main organ functions, namely intestinal calcium absorption, bone calcium resorption, and renal calcium excretion. Enhanced bioavailability thus results from a stimulation of calcium absorption and/or a decrease of calcium secretion at the intestinal level, a decrease of calcium resorption and/or an increase of calcium accretion at the skeletal level, a decrease of glomerular calcium filtration and/or an increase in tubular calcium reabsorption at the kidney level, or a combination of two or more of these processes involved in the metabolism of calcium by the human organism.

According to Norman [1], the following schematic model of calcium metabolism can be presented for the average adult male having a daily intake of 1.0 g calcium and of 0.8 g phosphorus (Fig. 1): In addition to the calcium ingested in the diet, approximately 600 to 700 mg are added to the intestinal contents via intestinal secretions. Since in this situation only a total amount of approximately 700 mg calcium (roughly 40%) is absorbed across the intestinal epithelium and passes into the blood stream, the remaining 900 to 1,000 mg are left in the gut lumen to be excreted in the feces. The calcium ions that have been absorbed enter a small extracellular pool that is in constant and rapid exchange with the calcium present in intracellular fluids and certain compartments of bone. Moreover, the extracellular calcium is

From INSERM U. 90, Département de Néphrologie, Hôpital Necker, Paris, France.

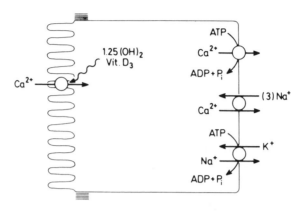

Fig. 1. Schematic model of calcium and phosphorus metabolism in an adult man having a calcium intake of 1.0 g/day and a phosphorus intake of 0.8 g/day. All numerical values are shown in milligrams per day. All entries relating to phosphate are calculated as phosphorus. (Reproduction from Norman, Vitamin D: The calcium homeostatic steroid hormone, chap. 10. "Intestinal Effects of Vitamin D." New York: Academic Press, 1979.)

constantly filtered at the glomerular level and reabsorbed by the kidney tubules. Thus, the entire extracellular pool of calcium turns over between 40 and 50 times a day. The magnitude of the daily glomerular filtration of calcium is as high as 10,000 mg. Fortunately, the renal tubular reabsorption of the ion is so efficient (97 to 99% of the ultrafiltered load) that under normal circumstances only between 100 and 300 mg is lost daily by urinary excretion. The extracellular pool of calcium consists of a vascular and an extravascular pool. In the former, calcium is present in different physical forms including ionized, protein-bound, and a small fraction of unbound, unionized calcium. The bone pool can be schematically subdivided into a "readily exchangeable" and a "slowly exchangeable" pool. The term "readily exchangeable" corresponds to a functional, not to an anatomical definition. It simply represents that fraction of calcium in bone which is in rapid equilibrium with the extracellular calcium, namely on a minute-to-minute exchange basis. Thus, of the total bone calcium of 1,000 to 1,200 g in a 70-kg man, approximately 0.4%, or 4,000 mg, is present in the "readily exchangeable" pool compartment.

A tight homeostatic regulation of plasma-ionized calcium concentration, and hence indirectly of the extracellular pool, is mainly guaranteed by three hormonal systems: parathyroid hormone, 1,25 diOH vitamin D3 (calcitriol) which is the most active vitamin D metabolite, and to a lesser degree, calcitonin. In addition to these hormonal regulations, a variety of other factors is also involved in the metabolism of calcium. They may all play a more or less important role in calcium homeostasis.

TABLE 1. Factors Able to Enhance the Efficiency of Intestinal Calcium Absorption

1,25-dihydroxyvitamin D3 (calcitriol)
Luminal-ionized calcium concentration
Sodium
Solvent drag
Milk products (lactose, casein, and derived phosphopeptides)
Calcium citrate

In terms of dietary and drug intervention aiming at an increased bioavailability of calcium, the major impact lies at the level of the intestine and bone. In the following presentation, our considerations will mainly focus on factors involved in intestinal calcium absorption which could have an influence on the bioavailability of the ion in normal healthy adults in terms of a more positive—or a more negative—balance. In addition to dietary factors, the nutritional and metabolic state of the host—such as calcium and vitamin D status, age, pregnancy, and lactation—plays of course a major role in the bioavailability and the balance of calcium. In the long run, this balance is essentially reflected by the level of bone calcium, which constitutes by far the most important reservoir of the ion (the "calcium bank" of the body).

FACTORS THAT ENHANCE CALCIUM BIOAVAILABILITY VIA INTESTINAL CALCIUM ABSORPTION (TABLE 1)

A variety of hormonal and nonhormonal factors influences the intestinal absorption and secretion of calcium. Before addressing this issue in a more detailed fashion, a brief recall of our present state of knowledge concerning the mechanisms of intestinal calcium transport [2–5] appears appropriate (Fig. 2). The calcium ion leaves the gut lumen by entering the intestinal epithelium via the enterocyte's brush border membrane, down a steep electrochemical gradient favoring passive movement of calcium into the cell. The ion is then transported to the serosal side of the enterocyte through a still unknown mechanism. It is extruded from the cell via the basolateral membrane by at least two different mechanisms, namely the calcium ATPase pump on the one hand and Na/Ca exchange on the other. This transport step is linked to a source of energy derived from cellular processes. Whether in addition to the transcellular pathway, the paracellular route of transport is also operative for calcium absorption to any significant extent remains an open question at present. As to the reverse transport of the ion from the serosal to the mucosal side of the intestine, namely calcium secretion, the preferred (or unique?) pathway appears to be the paracellular route. The driving forces for calcium movement along these paths may derive from

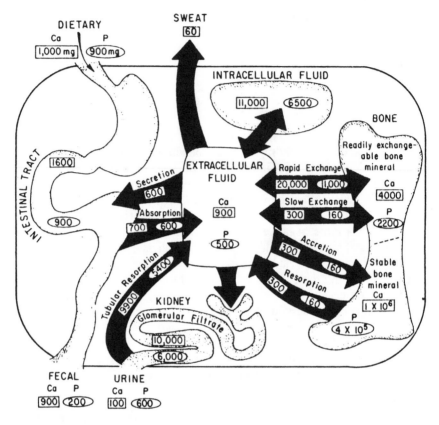

Fig. 2. Model for transcellular transport of calcium in small intestine. Calcium is taken up by the enterocyte across the brush border membrane. The entry step is facilitated by 1,25(OH)$_2$ vit. D3 (calcitriol). The extension step across the basolateral membrane involves active transport mechanisms involving Ca^{2+}-ATPase and/or calcium-sodium exchange. (Reproduced from Murer and Hildmann, *American Journal Physiology* 240:G409–G416, 1981.)

electrochemical potential gradients, energy-dependent cellular processes, solvent drag, or hydrostatic forces.

It must also be pointed out that techniques available for measuring intestinal calcium transport are of variable value. Results obtained with different methods must always be interpreted with caution and with the knowledge of their limitations. Thus, in vitro studies performed with isolated gut segments, cells or subcellular fractions may often result in valuable information on transport mechanisms, but may be of only limited value for clinical purposes. On the other hand, studies conducted in vivo may be subjected to large errors because of the complexity of the explored organism and its regulatory systems. They may in addition be subjected to criticisms because artificial investigation procedures often differ from normal situations. Thus, the intestinal perfusion in situ using the triple lumen tube represents a particular, acute and unphysiological situation from which extrapolations to the absorption of calcium on a day-to-day basis can be made only with extreme caution; inaccuracies in the collection of fecal samples will cause large errors in estimates of calcium absorption using the balance technique; and the use of calcium isotopes will lead to the determination of the fractional absorption of calcium administered in a form, a quantity, and/or a way different from that ingested with the usual diet. One should always have this caution in mind before extrapolating too rapidly from a given experimental result of intestinal calcium transport to usual dietary conditions in vivo.

Calcitriol

The main hormonal regulator of intestinal calcium transport is calcitriol, the active metabolite of vitamin D [2–5]. Calcitriol enhances the entry step across the brush border membrane, probably due to several mechanisms including the enhanced formation and/or accumulation of proteins having a high affinity for the calcium ion such as IMCAL [6] and calmodulin [7] at the site of this membrane. Calcitriol could in addition open calcium channels across the brush border membrane in a still unknown manner. These vitamin D dependent channels, if present, appear to be different from those blocked by calcium channel blockers such as verapamil or nitrendipine, at least at the level of the cecum [8]. Within the cytoplasm of the enterocyte, calcitriol enhances the formation of calcium-binding protein, CaBP [4], which must somehow be implicated in the capacity of the cell to accept calcium and to translocate it from the mucosal to the serosal side. Whether this hormone participates also in the regulation of the exit step at the basolateral side of the enterocyte remains a matter of speculation. At least one study [9] reported a stimulating effect of calcitriol on calcium-ATPase, which is thought to actively extrude the calcium ion to the serosal side against a steep electrochemical gradient. In addition to its well-known mode of action as a steroid hormone, namely via genomic nuclear activation [10], calcitriol has been shown more recently to exert also more direct effects on the enterocyte's membrane permeability to calcium, independent of de novo protein synthesis [11,12].

Calcitriol stimulates the active (or "mediated") component of intestinal calcium transport in a dose-dependent, saturable manner and with decreasing efficiency from the duodenum to the ileum and the colon. The stimulation of active transport observed in the aged human organism [13]—as well as in the aged animal organism [14]—in response to a given dose of calcitriol is much less pronounced than that of the younger organism. This indicates that the magnitude of active calcium transport by the gut declines with increasing age.

Luminal Calcium Concentration

The passive component of intestinal calcium transport is a direct function of the luminal calcium concentration [15,16], at least for concentrations higher than Kt, which is the medium calcium concentration at half maximal calcium flux (1/2 V_{max}). Passive calcitriol-independent calcium mucosal-to-serosal movement increases therefore linearly as luminal calcium concentrations exceed Kt. The pathway of the nonsaturable component is not understood. A paracellular pathway has been proposed [17] and cannot be excluded. Quantitatively, the nonsaturable component seems similar in the duodenum, jejunum, and ileum and seems unaffected by the level of oral calcium intake, at least in experimental animals [18]. The nonsaturable component decreases at an early age and at the same rate at which the saturable component increases [14]. In the older growing animal, the calcitriol-regulatable, saturable system of calcium absorption becomes increasingly predominant. In the old animal, a reversal occurs. Thus, the older organism is much more dependent than the younger one on an appropriate dietary intake of calcium in order to assure adequate calcium absorption rates.

Sodium

The sodium ion may theoretically alter calcium absorption at two key steps, namely the luminal and the serosal side of the enterocyte. Whereas there is no firm evidence for a direct interaction of sodium with calcium at the brush border membrane site, indirect effects through alterations in transmembrane potential have been observed [5]. Thus, calcium influx was decreased in experiments where sodium transport was enhanced by glucose [19] whereas calcium influx was increased in an incubation milieu where the sodium ion was replaced by mannitol [20]. Calcium extrusion across the basolateral membrane may be accomplished in part by sodium-calcium exchange. This may explain the reduction in duodenal calcium transport in sodium-free serosal medium [20]. Moreover, the importance of sodium-calcium exchange may vary by intestinal region, since sodium replacement by choline increased ileal but decreased cecal net absorption of calcium [5]. Ouabain, like sodium replacement, reduces net calcium absorption in the cecum but not in other intestinal segments, an effect attenuated by a diet rich in calcium [21]. Oral sodium chloride loading in healthy volunteers was shown to increase calcium absorption as measured by the 47-Ca absorption test [22]. However, since the increased absorption was not accompanied by a detectable change in calcium balance, a compensatory enhancement of calcium secretion must have occurred.

Solvent Drag

Increasing net water absorption in in vivo perfused segments of rat ileum with actively transported sugars such as glucose or galactose leads to concomitant increases in the absorption of calcium, independent of vitamin D [23]. Similar findings were reported for the human jejunum using the triple-lumen tube perfusion technique [24]. The glucose-stimulated water absorption led to an increase in luminal calcium concentration. However, when luminal calcium was maintained constant, calcium absorption was dissociated from water movement. These findings suggest that water absorption could increase the absorption of calcium by either the coupling of solute (calcium) and solvent flow or by changing either diffusive or active transport as a result of volume flow-dependent changes in calcium concentration at the brush-border surface [5].

Lactose

Oral lactose increases serum calcium, helps to replete bone mineral content, and restores the calcemic respone to parathyroid extract [25]. These beneficial effects of oral lactose appear to result from increased intestinal calcium absorption [26,27]. Lactose in the diet [28], either by addition of lactose to solutions instilled into in situ ligated loops [18] or in vitro addition of the disaccharide to medium bathing intestinal gut segments or sacs [8,29,30], enhances calcium absorption, regardless of the vitamin D status of the animal. However, the effect of lactose in vitro appears to be additive to that of vitamin D, as the incremental increase in net calcium transport by the disaccharide was greater in intestinal tissue from calcitriol-treated rats [8]. The direct stimulatory action of lactose, although not confined to the ileum [30], appears to be located mainly at the distal part of the small intestine. As lactose fails to undergo hydrolysis in the duodenum and jejunum, large quantities are delivered to the ileum where the disaccharide reduces luminal sodium content to maintain fluid isosmotic with plasma [5]. Isosmotic replacement of sodium with lactose, as with choline, creates no transepithelial gradients, but local intraepithelial gradients—perhaps across the tight junction—could occur and thereby induce local fluid shifts leading to an increased calcium concentration at the luminal surface [29]. It must, however, be recognized that the cellular basis for lactose stimulation of calcium transport remains unknown at present.

As to the effect of lactose on the bioavailability of calcium, dietary lactose has been reported to increase fractional absorption, decrease fecal calcium and increase urinary calcium in rats [31], but precise balance studies have not been performed in this experimental study to determine the potential effect of lactose on calcium retention. In another experimental study [32], dietary lactose administered to rats during four weeks led to an increase in bone ash but not in bone breaking strength parameters. In the same report, lactose administered to pigs during 70 days did not result in an improvement of skeletal resistance to physical stress. In other one-day balance studies [33], dietary lactose enhanced the femoral deposition of 45-calcium. Finally, lactose added to the normal calcium intake of four human volunteers proved to increase calcium retention [34].

The potentially negative effect of lactase deficiency, and hence malabsorption of lactose, on intestinal calcium transport is still controversial [35–37]. In one human study by Cochet et al. [35], oral lactose increased the fraction of calcium absorbed by normal subjects but decreased that absorbed by lactase-deficient individuals during the first 60 min after oral calcium intake. Two to seven hr after lactose ingestion calcium absorption rates were slightly increased in lactase-deficient, but heavily increased in normal subjects, possibly due to a stimulation of calcium transport by lactose appearing in the distal small intestine. The overall effect of lactose on total fractional absorption of calcium was therefore positive in normal volunteers but negative in lactase-deficient subjects. A direct relation was found in a more recent study by Pacifici et al. [36] between declining calcium absorption and decreasing lactase activity in postmenopausal women with osteoporosis and normal lactose tolerance. These authors claimed that varying degrees of relative deficiencies in intestinal lactase deficiency might contribute to the graded decrease in calcium absorption observed in the aging population. However, since this study was based on only a small population sample, more ample investigations are clearly required before such a relationship can be considered to be firmly established. Other authors [37] have claimed recently that malabsorption of lactose does not seem to impair the absorption of calcium from milk but no experimental arguments were provided.

Casein and Derived Phosphopeptides

The precise role of casein and derived products on calcium bioavailability is still unclear. One early study [38] in rats reached the conclusion that feeding casein, as compared to soybean as the dietary protein source, together with various amounts of added calcium carbonate resulted in no difference in femoral calcium retention. However, the time of administration of only four weeks may have been too short to detect such a difference. Moreover, no information was provided on the initial weight of the animals used. Wilson and Schedl [39] examined the effect of dietary casein versus fibrin on calcium balance in rats. They found a more positive balance with casein in rats submitted to a very low calcium intake (0.02%) whereas no difference in balance existed in rats on a normal calcium intake (1.2%). In contrast to the findings in vivo, the in vitro absorption of calcium using the duodenal sac technique was higher in fibrin than in casein fed animals on low calcium intake. This could reflect an adequate response of the intestinal mucosa to achieve a more positive calcium balance. Lee et al. [40] administered casein or various protein diets other than casein to rats and examined thereafter the physical state of calcium contained in the small intestinal tract. They observed that 2.5 hr after ingestion, the amounts of soluble calcium was higher in animals fed the casein diet than in those fed egg albumin, soybean protein, or an amino acid mixture. In subsequent experiments in rats [41], these authors were able to demonstrate an increase in net calcium absorption from in situ ligated intestinal loops after feeding of casein, as compared to other protein sources. They hypothesized that the tryptic digestion of casein generated phosphopeptides having the capacity of increasing the amount of soluble calcium in the intestinal lumen by preventing the formation of insoluble calcium phosphate complexes. Such an hypothesis had already been proposed previously by Mykkänen and Wasserman [42] based on experimental studies in chicks. These authors introduced tryptic hydrolysates of casein into in situ ligated intestinal loops and found an increase in calcium absorption, as compared to that observed in the presence of peptides derived from albumin. In addition, they were able to show a similar increase of calcium transport to occur in everted gut sacs that were exposed to casein-derived phosphopeptides.

An exciting recent development in this field is the observation that opiatelike peptides, so-called β-casomorphins, have been described to occur in enzymatic digests of milk casein. These opioid peptides are able to decrease intestinal short-circuit current and to stimulate intestinal sodium and chloride transport, as has been demonstrated in isolated segments of rabbit ileum [43]. At our knowledge, no studies have been reported thus far concerning the potential effects of either natural or synthetic β-casomorphins on intestinal calcium transport.

Unprocessed and Processed Milk

Only a limited number of investigations has been devoted to the bioavailability of calcium from entire dairy products which are the most important source of calcium in the diet of Western countries. In studies performed in weaning rats, Wong and LaCroix [44] observed an increase of femur calcium content in response to nonfat dry milk, yogurt, and rennet-precipitated casein by 18%, 9% and 44%, respectively as compared to a nondairy protein source. The animals were receiving the respective dairy sources of protein during three weeks before sacrifice. Partridge [45] compared the effects of two protein diets on calcium metabolism in young pigs. This author found that the administration of skim milk, as compared to

TABLE 2. Factors Able to Diminish the Efficiency of Intestinal Calcium Absorption or to Modify Calcium Secretion

Inhibition of absorption
  Phosphorus
  Plant components (dietary fiber)
  Fat
  Alcohol
  Hormones (calcitonin, glucocorticoids, thyroxin)
  Genetic influences (spontaneously hypertensive rat)
  Drugs (thiazide diuretics, phenothiazines)

Change of secretion
  Extracellular fluid and plasma volume expansion (sodium load)
  Low-calcium diet
  Hormones (somatostatin)

soybean, led to a higher rate of intestinal calcium absorption and a greater body calcium retention.

Calcium Citrate

Very recently, attention has been drawn to the possibly important role that the anion of ingested calcium salts could play in the bioavailability of the cation, calcium. Thus, two reports [46,47] claimed a possible superiority of the water-soluble calcium citrate over the water-insoluble calcium carbonate in enhancing intestinal calcium absorption. However, whereas Nicar and Pak [46] found such an effect in normal volunteers, Recker [47] observed a greater amount of absorbed calcium with citrate as the anion only in patients with achlorhydria, but not in healthy subjects. On closer scrutiny it appears that marked methodological differences between the two studies could at least partially explain the discrepancy of their results in normal subjects. In the former study, the dose of cold calcium used was 4-fold higher, and the analyzing method of intestinal calcium absorption was rather indirect (urinary calcium excretion), whereas calcium absorption was more directly evaluated in the latter study (fractional absorption method using 45-Ca). Although it seems logical to presume that gastric acidity and acid secretion play a major role in the absorption of calcium from food and calcium salts, this assumption has recently been disproved by studies in healthy volunteers and patients with pernicious anemia [48]. Since calcium absorbed from calcium carbonate in the total absence of gastric acid must have been solubilized prior to absorption, it can be hypothesized that the solubilization was achieved through acid secretion by the enterocytes, through the fixed negative surface charge of these cells, or through the effect of biliary and pancreatic secretions [48].

An interesting additional aspect of the use of calcium citrate lies in the observation that an enhanced urinary excretion of citrate is associated with an augmented inhibitory activity against calcium oxalate crystallization [49] and hence a decreased propensity for the formation of kidney stones in subjects receiving increased oral loads of calcium. The possible advantage of calcium citrate over calcium carbonate clearly deserves more investigation, in terms of calcium retention in the organism and long-term tolerance, before its general acceptance.

FACTORS ABLE TO INHIBIT CALCIUM BIOAVAILABILITY VIA MODIFYING INTESTINAL CALCIUM ABSORPTION OR SECRETION

Inhibition of Calcium Absorption

Many factors including dietary components, hormones and drugs may interfere with the intestinal absorption of calcium (Table 2).

Phosphorus

The amount and the type of phosphorus present in the intestinal lumen could play a role in vivo, but this issue is highly controversial. Thus in animals, continuous feeding of a high phosphorus intake, or a high phosphorus to calcium ratio, results in bone resorption secondary to hyperparathyroidism. Perhaps for this reason, it is generally assumed that a high phosphorus to calcium ratio may have a deleterious effect on intestinal calcium absorption in humans [50]. However, Spencer et al. [51] showed in balance studies in healthy male volunteers that no interference of a high phosphorus intake (up to 2,000 mg/day) occurred with the calcium absorbed by the gut, irrespective of the calcium intake which varied by a factor of 10. Although not mentioned by the authors, fecal calcium did increase (not significantly) as phosphorus intake increased, and this was accompanied by a significant decrease in urinary calcium [50]. Moreover, it must be pointed out here that balance studies are inappropriate to detect small changes in calcium absorption. Since the phosphate salt used by Spencer et al. was sodium glycerophosphate, it may also be argued that interference with calcium absorption may be particularly low with this form of phosphate. In contrast, phosphorus present in the lumen in the form of phytate is known to form an unabsorbable calcium phytate complex and thus to interfere with calcium absorption [50,52]. The independence of calcium absorption from dietary phosphorus level was however also reported in infants by Barltrop et al. [53]. In in vitro experiments using isolated intestinal gut sacs or segments, an independence of the luminal transport step for calcium from that for phosphate has generally been observed in more recent studies, in contrast to a previously held theory, even though the absorptive fluxes of both ion species are stimulated by vitamin

D [5]. Taken together, there is not much evidence to suggest that dietary phosphorus plays an important inhibitory role in the intestinal absorption of calcium, unless the phosphorus is present in the form of phytate.

Plant Components

It has long been known that feeding whole wheat products to humans can result in negative calcium balance [50]. Cummings et al. [54] observed that a marked increase of dietary fiber intake in their subjects studied led to a considerable reduction in calcium balance. In addition to the negative effect of phytate (see above), fiber itself appears to impair calcium absorption [55–57]. Attempts to identify the components of fiber that could inhibit calcium absorption have led to the incrimination of various materials including cellulose [58,59], uronic acid [60], sodium alginate, a polysaccharide extracted from seaweed [61], and oxalate [62,63]. Ascorbic acid has been reported to enhance calcium absorption, but the concomitantly observed stimulation of urinary calcium excretion has left the calcium balance unchanged [64].

Fat

The effect of dietary fat on calcium absorption is far from being firmly established. In the healthy adult, variations of ingested fat (butter) from 1 to 32% of the diet did not change calcium balance [65]. Even in steatorrhea, where intestinal calcium absorption has been found to be reduced by some authors [66, 67], it has been reported to be unchanged by others [68,69]. An interaction can occur due to the precipitation of calcium with fatty acids and the formation of insoluble soap in the gut lumen. The availability of calcium from these soaps apparently diminishes with increasing chain length and increasing saturation of fatty acids [70]. Interestingly, the inhibitory effect of added dietary calcium on colonic epithelial-cell proliferation in subjects at high risk of colon cancer has recently been attributed to an interaction between dietary calcium and luminal fatty acids [71], even though other mechanisms should also be tentatively envisaged [72].

Alcohol

Chronic alcoholism can impair the intestinal absorption of calcium as a result of steatorrhea with subsequent decrease in vitamin D absorption and possibly impaired vitamin hydroxylation by the cirrhotic liver [73]. In addition, chronic alcoholism may alter calcium intake by decreasing appetite and displacing calcium-rich foods in the diet [74]. In the experimental animal, intestinal calcium absorption can also be decreased by oral alcohol ingestion in the absence of vitamin D deficiency [75], in line with a direct toxic effect of ethanol on the intestinal mucosa [76].

Hormones

The action of calcitonin on intestinal calcium transport is controversial. Whereas some authors found no effect of this peptide hormone on calcium transport across rat ileum in vitro [77], others found an inhibition of calcium absorption in the isolated vascularly perfused intestine using physiological doses of calcitonin [78].

An interference of glucocorticoids with intestinal calcium absorption has been demonstrated. Thus, cortisone treatment inhibits active calcium transport in the proximal, but not the distal, small intestine [79]. In the colon, however, glucocorticoid-treated rats exhibit an increased transport of calcium [80]. The situation is more complex in vivo since glucocorticoids stimulate the absorption of sodium and water, thereby resulting in an increase in the passive transport of calcium [81]. Thus, depending upon the region of intestine under consideration and the prevailing situation of water movement, passive calcium absorption may overcome the inhibitory effect of glucocorticoids on active transport in the proximal small intestine.

The thyroid status could also be of importance since thyroxin has been shown to exert a direct inhibitory effect on intestinal calcium absorption [82], and calcium malabsorption may occur in patients with hyperthyroidism [83,84].

Genetic Influences

The spontaneously hypertensive rat (SHR) represents an experimental model of genetically predetermined hypertension associated with a variety of anomalies of calcium metabolism. In recent personal studies in vitro [85,86], we have been able to document using the Ussing chamber model that the duodenal calcium absorption of the SHR is decreased as compared to it genetic control, the WKY rat. The decrease is limited to the lumen-to-serosa component of transport, is associated with a diminished circulating level of calcitriol, and can be corrected upon exogenous administration of the hormone.

Drugs

Several drugs have been shown to influence calcium absorption. Thus, thiazide diuretics and analogous molecules such as chlorthalidone and hydrochlorothiazide have been recently demonstrated to reduce intestinal calcium absorption in experimental animals [87] and in women with postmenopausal osteoporosis [88]. The inhibitor of calmodulin-dependent, calcium-activated ATPase, trifluoroperazine has also been shown to reduce the intestinal transport of calcium directed from the mucosa to the serosa [89].

Changes of Calcium Secretion (Table 2)

The information available regarding calcium secretion is scarce. An increase in blood ionized calcium concentration may alter the transmucosal calcium gradient and hence stimulate calcium secretion [5]. Increased hydrostatic pressure due to extracellular fluid [90] or plasma volume [91] expansion also favors calcium secretion. An increased oral sodium chloride load also leads to increased calcium secretion [22], representing probably a compensatory mechanism in response to the increased calcium absorption observed under such conditions.

Low calcium diet reduces the plasma-to-lumen movement of calcium during in situ perfusion of loops of rat ileum [92], but ileal calcium transport in the luminal direction under short-circuited conditions in vitro is not altered by dietary calcium restriction or calcitriol [17,29,93].

Somatostatin addition in vitro stimulates serosal-to-mucosal calcium movement in ileum and descending colon [94], possibly via a direct action on calcium secretion [95] since the hormone stimulates sodium and water absorption.

CONCLUSIONS

A great number of factors influence the bioavailability of calcium through changes of the intestinal absorption of calcium. Besides factors related to the host status such as age, pregnancy and lactation, and metabolic as well as hormonal changes related to disease, nutritional factors clearly play an important role. The relative importance of the various components of the diet in the bioavailability and body retention of calcium in the long run is still difficult to assess and may be different from one subject to the other, from one geographical area to another, and from one time period to another with changing dietary habits and environmental conditions.

Clearly, an adequate amount of regularly ingested calcium is of utmost importance to avoid a negative calcium balance. The precise amount of calcium required may be more or less elevated depending on the physical status and the dietary habits of each subject.

REFERENCES

1. Norman AW (1979):Vitamin D metabolism and calcium absorption. Am J Med 67: 989–998.
2. Bikle DD, Morrissey RL, Zolock DT, Rasmussen H (1981):The intestinal response to vitamin D. Rev Physiol Biochem Pharmacol 89:63–142.
3. Norman AW, Putkey JA, Nemere I (1982):Intestinal calcium transport: pleiotropic effects mediated by vitamin D. Fed Proc 41:78–83.

4. Wasserman RH, Fullmer CS (1983):Calcium transport proteins, calcium absorption, and vitamin D. Ann Rev Physiol 45:375–390.

5. Favus MJ (1985):Factors that influence absorption and secretion of calcium in the small intestine and colon. Am J Physiol 248:G147–G157.

6. Kowarski S, Schachter D (1980):Intestinal membrane calcium-binding protein, a vitamin D dependent membrane protein component of the intestinal calcium transport mechanism. J Biol Chem 255:10834–10840.

7. Bikle DD, Munson S (1985):1,25-dihydroxyvitamin D increases calmodulin binding to specific proteins in the chick duodenal brush border membrane. J Clin Invest 76:2312–2316.

8. Favus MJ, Angeid-Backman E (1985):Effects of $1,25(OH)_2D_3$ and calcium channel blockers on cecal calcium transport in the rat. Am J Physiol 248:G676–G681.

9. Ghijsen WEJM, van Os CH (1982):1,25-dihydroxyvitamin D3 regulates ATP-dependent calcium transport in basolateral membranes of rat small intestine. Biochim Biophys Acta 689:170–172.

10. DeLuca HF, Schnoes HK (1983):Vitamin D: recent advances. Ann Rev Biochem 52:411–439.

11. Bikle DD, Zolock DT, Morrissey RL, Herman RH (1978):Independence of 1,25-dihydroxyvitamin D-mediated calcium transport from de novo RNA and protein synthesis. J Biol Chem 253:484–488.

12. Rasmussen H, Matsumoto T, Fontaine O, Goodman DBP (1982):Role of changes in membrane lipid structure in the action of 1,25-dihydroxyvitamin D3. Fed Proc 41:72–77.

13. Ireland P, Fordtran JS (1973):Effect of dietary calcium and age on jejunal calcium absorption in humans studied by intestinal perfusion. J Clin Invest 52:2672–2681.

14. Pansu D, Bellaton C, Bronner F (1983):Developmental changes in the mechanisms of duodenal calcium transport in the rat. Am J Physiol 244:G20–G26.

15. Pansu D, Bellaton C, Roche C, Bronner F (1983):Duodenal and ileal calcium absorption in the rat and effects of vitamin D. Am J Physiol 244:G695–G700.

16. Schedl HP, Wilson HD (1985):Calcium uptake by intestinal brush border membrane vesicles. Comparison with in vivo calcium transport. J Clin Invest 76:1871–1878.

17. Nellans HN, Kimberg DV (1979):Anomalous secretion of calcium in rat ileum:role of the paracellular pathway. Am J Physiol 236:E473–E481.

18. Pansu D, Bellaton C, Bronner F (1981):The effect of calcium intake on the saturable and nonsaturable components of duodenal calcium transport. Am J Physiol 240:G32–G37.

19. Patrick G, Sterling C (1973):The dependence of calcium influx into rat intestine on sugar and alkali metals. Arch Int Physiol Biochem 81:453–467.

20. Martin DL, De Luca HF (1969):Influence of sodium on calcium transport by rat small intestine. Am J Physiol 216:1351–1359.

21. Nellans HN, Goldsmith RS (1981):Transepithelial calcium transport by rat cecum: high-efficiency absorptive site. Am J Physiol 240:G424–G431.

22. Meyer WJ III, Transbol I, Bartter FC, Delea C (1976):Control of calcium absorption: effect of sodium chloride loading and depletion. Metabolism 25:989–993.

23. Behar J, Kerstein MD (1976):Intestinal calcium absorption: differences in transport between duodenum and ileum. Am J Physiol 230:1255–1260.

24. Norman DA, Morawski SG, Fordtran JS (1980):Influence of glucose, fructose, and water movement on calcium absorption in the jejunum. Gastroenterology 78:22–25.

25. Au WYW, Raisz LG (1967):Restoration of parathyroid responsiveness in vitamin D-deficient rats by parenteral calcium or dietary lactose. J Clin Invest 46:1572–1577.

26. Lengemann FW, Comar CL (1961):Distribution of absorbed strontium-85 and calcium-45 as influenced by lactose. Am J Physiol 200:1051–1054.

27. Chang YO, Hagstedt DM (1964):Lactose and calcium transport in gut sacs. J Nutr 82: 297–300.

28. Lengemann FW, Wasserman RH, Comar CL (1959):Studies on the enhancement of radiocalcium and radiostrontium absorption by lactose in the rat. J Nutr 68:443–456.

29. Favus MJ, Angeid-Backman E (1984):Effects of lactose on calcium absorption and secretion by rat ileum. Am J Physiol 246:G281–G285.

30. Armbrecht HJ, Wasserman RH (1976):Enhancement of Ca^{++} uptake by lactose in the rat small intestine. J Nutr 106:1265–1271.

31. Leichter J, Tolensky AF (1975):Effect of dietary lactose on the absorption of protein, fat and calcium in the postweaning rat. Am J Clin Nutr 28:238–241.

32. Moser RL, Peo ER, Crensgaw TD, Cunningham PJ (1980):Effect of dietary lactose on gain, feed conversion, blood, bone and intestinal parameters in postweaning rats and swine. J Animal Sci 51:89–99.

33. Sato R, Noguchi T, Naito H (1983):Effect of lactose on calcium absorption from the rat small intestine with a non-flushed ligated loop. J Nutr Sci Vitaminol 29:365–373.

34. Condon JR, Nassim JR, Millard FJC, Hilbe A, Stainthorpe EM (1970):Calcium and phosphorus metabolism in relation to lactose tolerance. Lancet 1:1027–1029.

35. Cochet B, Jung A, Griessen M, Bartholdi P, Schaller P, Donath A (1983):Effects of lactose on intestinal calcium absorption in normal and lactase-deficient subjects. Gastroenterology 84:935–940.

36. Pacifici R, Droke D, Avioli LV (1985):Intestinal lactase activity and calcium absorption in the aging female with osteoporosis. Calcif Tissue Int 37:101–102.

37. Newcomer AD, McGill DB (1984):Clinical importance of lactase deficiency. N Engl J Med 310:42–43.

38. Forbes RM, Weingartner KE, Parker HM, Bell RR, Erdman JW Jr (1979):Bioavailability to rats of zinc, magnesium and calcium in casein-, egg- and soy protein-containing diets. J Nutr 109:1652–1660.

39. Wilson HD, Schedl HP (1981):Effects of casein and fibrin on calcium absorption and calcium homeostasis in the rat. Dig Dis Sci 26:237–241.

40. Lee YS, Noguchi T, Naito H (1980):Phosphopeptides and soluble calcium in the small intestine of rats given a casein diet. Br J Nutr 43:457–467.

41. Lee YS, Noguchi T, Naito H (1983):Intestinal absorption of calcium in rats given diets containing casein or amino acid mixture: the role of casein phosphopeptides. Br J Nutr 49:67–76.

42. Mykkänen HM, Wasserman RH (1980):Enhanced absorption of calcium by casein phosphopeptides in rachitic and normal chicks. J Nutr 110:2141–2148.

43. Hautefeuille M, Brantl V, Dumontier AM, Desjeux JF (1986):In vitro effects of β-casomorphins on ion transport in rabbit ileum. Am J Physiol 250:G92–G97.

44. Wong NP, LaCroix DE (1980):Biological availability of calcium in dairy products. Nutr Rep Internat 21:673–680.

45. Partridge IG (1981):A comparison of defluorinated rock phosphate and dicalcium phosphate, in diets containing either skim milk powder or soya bean meal as the main protein supplement, for early-weaned pigs. Anim Prod 32:67–73.

46. Nicar MJ, Pak CYC (1985):Calcium bioavailability from calcium carbonate and calcium citrate. J Clin Endocrinol Metab 61:391–393.

47. Recker RR (1985):Calcium absorption and achlorhydria. N Engl J Med 313:70–73.

48. Bo-Linn GW, Davis GR, Buddrus DJ, Morawski SG, Santa Ana C, Fordtran JS (1984):An evaluation of the importance of gastric acid secretion in the absorption of dietary calcium. J Clin Invest 73:640–647.

49. Harvey JA, Zobitz MM, Pak CYC (1985):Reduced propensity for the crystallization of

calcium oxalate in urine resulting from induced hypercalciuria of calcium supplementation. J Clin Endocrinol Metab 61:1223–1225.

50. Allen LH (1982):Calcium bioavailability and absorption: a review. Am J Clin Nutr 35: 783–808.

51. Spencer H, Kramer L, Osis D, Norris C (1978):Effect of phosphorus on the absorption of calcium and on calcium balance in man. J Nutr 108:447–457.

52. Pointillart A, Fontaine N, Thomasset M, Jay ME (1985):Phosphorus utilization, intestinal phosphatases and hormonal control of calcium metabolism in pigs fed phytic phosphorus: soyabean or rapeseed diets. Nutr Rep Internat 32:155–167.

53. Barltrop D, Mole RH, Sutton A (1977):Absorption and endogenous faecal excretion of calcium by low birthweight infants on feed with varying contents of calcium and phosphate. Arch Dis Child 52:41–4953.

54. Cummings JH, Hill MJ, Houston H, Branch WJ, Jenkins DJA (1979):The effect of meat protein and dietary fiber on colonic function and metabolism. I. Changes in bowel habit, bile acid excretion and calcium absorption. Am J Clin Nutr 32:2086–2093.

55. Reinhold JG, Nasr K, Lahimgarzadeh A, Hedayati H (1973):Effects of purified phytate and phytate-rich bread upon metabolism of zinc, calcium, phosphorus and nitrogen in man. Lancet 1:283–288.

56. McCance RA, Widdowson EM (1942):Mineral balance on dephytinized bread. Am J Physiol 101:304–313.

57. Kelsay JL, Behall KM, Prather ES (1979):Effect of fiber from fruits and vegetables on metabolic responses of human subjects. II. Calcium, magnesium, iron, and silicon balances. Am J Clin Nutr 32:1876–1880.

58. Southgate DAT (1978):Dietary fiber:analyses and food sources. Am J Clin Nutr 31: 107–110.

59. Slavin JL, Marlett JA (1980):Influence of refined cellulose on human small bowel function and calcium and magnesium balance. Am J Clin Nutr 33:1932–1939.

60. James WPT, Branch WJ, Southgate DAT (1978):Calcium binding by dietary fiber. Lancet 1:638–639.

61. Harmuth-Hoene A-S, Schelenz R (1980):Effect of dietary fiber on mineral absorption in growing rats. J Nutr 110:1774–1784.

62. Bonner P, Hummel FC, Bates MF, Horton J, Hunscher HA, Macy IG (1938):The influence of a daily serving of spinach or its equivalent in oxalic acid upon the mineral utilization of children. J Pediatr 12:188–196.

63. Johnston FA, Macmillan TJ, Falconer GD (1952):Calcium retained by young women before and after adding spinach to the diet. J Am Diet Assoc 28:933–938.

64. Leichsenring JM, Norris LM, Halbert ML (1957):Effect of ascorbic acid and of orange juice on calcium and phosphorus metabolism of women. J Nutr 63:425–435.

65. Steggerda FR, Mitchell HH (1951):The calcium balance of adult human subjects on high- and low-fat (butter) diets. J Nutr 45:201–211.

66. Agnew JE, Holdsworth CD (1971):The effect of fat on calcium absorption from a mixed meal in normal subjects, patients with malabsorptive disease, and patients with a partial gastrectomy. Gut 12:973–977.

67. Hanna FM, Navarrette DA, Hsu FA (1970):Calcium-fatty acid absorption in term infants fed human milk and prepared formulas simulating human milk. Pediatrics 45:216–224.

68. Filer LJ Jr, Mattson FH, Fomon SJ (1970):Triglyceride configuration and fat absorption by the human infant. J Nutr 99:293–298.

69. Shaw JCL (1976):Evidence for defective skeletal mineralization in low-birthweight infants: the absorption of calcium and fat. Pediatrics 57:16–25.

70. Gacs G, Barltrop D (1977):Significance of Ca-soap formation for calcium absorption in the rat. Gut 18:64–68.
71. Lipkin M, Newmark H (1985):Effect of added dietary calcium on colonic epithelial-cell proliferation in subjects at high risk for familial colonic cancer. N Engl J Med 313:1381–1384.
72. Bresalier RS, Kim YS (1985):Diet and colon cancer. Putting the puzzle together. N Engl J Med 313:1413–1414.
73. Hepner GW, Roginsky M, Moo HF (1976):Abnormal vitamin D metabolism in patients with cirrhosis. Am J Dig Dis 21:527–532.
74. Spencer H, Kramer L, Osis D (1982):Factors contributing to calcium loss in aging. Am J Clin Nutr 36:776–787.
75. Krawitt EL (1975):Effect of ethanol ingestion on duodenal calcium transport. J Lab Clin Med 85:665–671.
76. Krawitt EL, Sampson HW, Katagiri CA (1975):Effect of 1,25-dihydroxy cholecalciferol on ethanol-mediated suppression of calcium absorption. Calcif Tissue Res 18:119–124.
77. Walling MW, Brasitus TA, Kimberg DV (1977):Effects of calcitonin and substance P on the transport of Ca, Na, and Cl across rat ileum in vitro. Gastroenterology 73:89–94.
78. Olson EB, DeLuca HF, Potts JT (1972):Calcitonin inhibition of vitamin D–induced intestinal calcium absorption. Endocrinology 90:151–157.
79. Kimberg DV, Baerg RD, Gerrshon E, Grandusius RT (1971):Effect of cortisone treatment on the active transport of calcium by the small intestine. J Clin Invest 50:1309–1321.
80. Lee DBN (1983):Unanticipated stimulatory action of glucocorticoids on epithelial calcium absorption: effect of dexamethasone on rat distal colon. J Clin Invest 71:322–328.
81. Yeh JK, Aloia JF (1986):Influence of glucocorticoids on calcium absorption in different segments of the rat intestine. Calcif Tissue Int 38:282–288.
82. Friedland JA, Williams GA, Bowser EN, Henderson WJ, Hoffeins E (1965):Effect of hyperthyroidism on intestinal absorption of calcium in the rat. Proc Soc Exp Biol Med 120:20–23.
83. Shafer RB, Gregory DH (1972):Calcium malabsorption in hyperthyroidism. Gastroenterology 63:235–239.
84. Peerenboom H, Keck E, Krüskremper HL, Strohmeyer G (1984):The defect of intestinal calcium transport in hyperthyroidism and its response to therapy. J Clin Endocrinol Metab 59:936–940.
85. McCarron DA, Lucas PA, Shneidman RJ, Lacour B, Drüeke T (1985):Blood pressure development of the spontaneously hypertensive rat following concurrent manipulations of dietary Ca^{2+} and Na^+: relation to intestinal Ca^{2+} fluxes. J Clin Invest 73:1147–1154.
86. Lucas PA, Brown RC, Drüeke T, Lacour B, Metz JA, McCarron DA (1986):Abnormal vitamin D metabolism, intestinal calcium transport, and bone calcium status in the spontaneously hypertensive rat compared with its genetic control. J Clin Invest 78:221–227.
87. Bushinsky DA, Favus MJ, Coe FL (1984):Mechanism of chronic hypercalciuria with chlorthalidone: reduced calcium absorption. Am J Physiol 247:F746–F752.
88. Sakhaee K, Nicar MJ, Glass K, Zerkwekh JE, Pak CYC (1984):Reduction in intestinal calcium absorption by hydrochlorothiazide in postmenopausal osteoporosis. J Clin Endocrinol Metab 59:1037–1043.
89. Favus MJ, Angeid-Backman E, Breyer MD, Coe FL (1983):Effects of trifluoperazine, ouabain, and ethacrynic acid on intestinal calcium transport. Am J Physiol 244:G111–G115.
90. Chanard J, Drüeke T, Pujade-Lauraine E, Lacour B, Funck-Brentano J-L (1976):Effects of saline loading on jejunal absorption of calcium, sodium, and water, and on parathyroid hormone secretion in the rat. Pflügers Arch 367:169–175.

91. Drüeke T, Chanard J, Lacour B, Pujade-Lauraine E, Funck-Brentano J-L (1978):Effects of hyperoncotic albumin on jejunal electrolyte and water absorption in the rat. Pflügers Arch 373:249–257.

92. Petith MM, Schedl HP (1976):Duodenal and ileal adaptation to dietary calcium restriction: in vivo studies in the rat. Am J Physiol 231:865–871.

93. Nellans HN, Kimberg DV (1978):Cellular and paracellular calcium transport in rat ileum: effects of dietary calcium. Am J Physiol 235:E726–E737.

94. Favus MJ, Berelowitz M, Coe FL (1981):Effects of somatostatin on intestinal calcium transport in the rat. Am J Physiol 241:G215–G221.

95. Evenson D, Hanssen KF, Berstad A (1978):Inhibition of intestinal calcium absorption by somatostatin in man. Metabolism 27:1345–1347.

Nutritional Factors in Hypertension
© *1990 Alan R. Liss, Inc., pages 175–197*

12   Calcium Intake and Blood Pressure: An Epidemiologic Perspective

William R. Harlan, M.D.
Lynne C. Harlan, Ph.D., M.P.H.

INTRODUCTION

Historically, sodium and potassium have been the dietary electrolytes of primary interest when determinants of blood pressure levels are considered. However, considerable recent attention has been directed to calcium as a factor both in the development and in the potential control of high blood pressure. There is ample physiological data that link cellular calcium movement to neuromuscular tone and potentially to physiological control of blood pressure [1]. At the cellular and subcellular levels, calcium concentrations and movement have major effects on neuromuscular excitability and could alter arterial smooth muscle tone. The recent clinical interest in dietary calcium and blood pressure does not derive from these physiologic associations but from numerous epidemiologic observations and from several intervention trials. These epidemiologic studies indicate that there is an inverse relationship between calcium intake, both dietary and supplemental, and blood pressure. Moreover, the successful use of calcium (slow channel) blockers in the treatment of hypertension and of supplemental calcium have highlighted the potential utility of this calcium–blood pressure connection in management of hypertension.

These considerations demand a careful assessment of the clinical evidence relating calcium intake to blood pressure. This chapter reviews the relation-

From the University of Michigan School of Medicine (W.R.H.) and the University of Michigan School of Public Health, G-1204 Towsley Center, University of Michigan Medical School, Ann Arbor, MI 48109.

ship from the perspective of epidemiological studies and of clinical intervention trials. The data support a consistent though not always strong relationship, and this association seems attributable to the calcium ion. The reasons for the variable strength of the association and for the cautious attribution to calcium are considered further. This review addresses the epidemiological and intervention trial evidence for an association and discusses the potential mechanisms for this association and the therapeutic implications to be drawn.

EPIDEMIOLOGICAL STUDIES

The case for a clinical association with high blood pressure is based on a rather extensive body of epidemiologic observations, largely derived from surveys of defined populations [2–14]. A rather extensive literature has developed over a brief period on the epidemiological relationship of dietary calcium to blood pressure [15]. In general, the analyses were performed a posteriori and used dietary information and blood pressure data collected without a prior hypothesis for an association. In some instances, collection of dietary data may have been less than optimal and the use of calcium or mineral supplements not assessed. An adequate assessment of the interaction of other nutritional components known to influence blood pressure or to interact with calcium (e.g., salt, potassium, alcohol, trace metals) requires good measurement of these components. The evaluation of these epidemiological studies requires an appreciation for the accuracy and representativeness of dietary intake and the acceptable tolerances for interpretation.

The current approaches for assessing dietary intake represent compromises between accuracy and representativeness of individual intake. The most accurate method is conceded to be the 24-hour dietary recall, but it represents only one day, and even that day's intake may be recalled with bias or poorly, particularly with respect to portion or size [16]. Also, food intake may be modified by the respondent in anticipation of the subsequent interview. Other assessments that aim at detecting the acknowledged daily variability of intake include longer periods of recall or use of diet diaries (3-day, 7-day, 30-day) or the use of semiquantitative frequency of food use over longer periods (3 months). These approaches provide a more representative estimate of the intake of major dietary constituents, albeit seasonally influenced, but quantification is limited, and less commonly ingested foods and beverages can be underreported. Moreover, levels of cooperation and reporting can vary differentially by socioeconomic status. The appropriate analytical approach to data using any of these methods is to aggregate data and to characterize average group intake, not to characterize individuals. The within-individual variability is too great to permit correlation of individual dietary intake with another finding. Therefore, group dietary data with adequate sample sizes are required for appropriate analysis and interpretation.

In contrast to many dietary constituents, calcium intake sources are relatively easily identified and comparatively well quantified using any of these methods. About 60 to 70 percent of calcium intake in the U.S. comes from dairy products, and a limited list of fairly simple questions can be used to assess intake [17]. The dairy sources are easily identified and have high calcium content. Additional significant sources of calcium include some nuts and green vegetables (kale, collards, broccoli, and spinach). While these latter sources may have been major sources for prehistoric man, the majority of persons do not consume sufficiently large amounts to make them an important calcium source [18]. Nevertheless, these sources can be identified easily with minimal probing. Therefore, the limited variety of significantly concentrated calcium sources simplifies quantification of intake.

The association between calcium and blood pressure has been found using only one simple measure of calcium—whole milk [5]. Dietary calcium can be easily measured with relatively few diet questions about dairy products. The majority of the dietary calcium in the U.S. is taken in the form of dairy products [19]. According to 1960 USDA figures, milk is the primary source of calcium [20]. Milk consumption in the U.S. has decreased and dairy product consumption, except for cheese, has been decreasing since 1965 [21]. A one-year study was conducted of 34 men and women aged 20 to 53 to determine the relationship between dietary intake of several nutrients, their excretion, and the balance maintained [18]. Daily diet diaries were kept for one year, and once each season duplicate food and beverages were collected for analyses. In addition, urine, feces, and blood samples were analyzed for content of these nutrients. Men consumed significantly more calcium than women. However, this was due to a greater intake of food. Intake of calcium was similar if calcium was expressed as mg Ca^{2+}/kcal or mg Ca^{2+}/kg body weight. Moreover, the investigators found no significant difference in calcium intake over the seasons, although there was variation in the excretion and balance. In a comparison of recorded and analyzed data, a simple correlation coefficient for calcium intake of 0.96 was found. This suggests that, at least in this sample, individual reported intake of calcium is very close to the actual measured intake.

The challenge is greater for most other dietary nutrients and particularly electrolytes, including sodium. Salt is ubiquitous in the diet of most industrialized societies and is "hidden" in the processing of foods so that it cannot be readily identified by consumers. Quantification requires an extensive and careful evaluation by trained nutritionists. Only studies that have directed special attention to assessing sodium and potassium can provide accurate intake data. Moreover, the discretionary use of salt added in cooking or at the table provides about one-third of customary intake, but is seldom assessed in the usual intake history. Even with special training, this source may be poorly quantified. Therefore, dietary data from most surveys are unlikely to provide a reliable assessment of sodium intake unless this was a planned focus of the study. This caveat is important in considering the data relating calcium to blood pressure, because sodium and potassium have associations with blood pressure and there are also hormonal and excretory interactions among calcium, sodium, and potassium. These interactions are discussed further under "Mechanisms." For review of the epidemiologic studies, the availability of intake estimates for sodium and potassium is noted, but the competing and interactive effects are not evaluated in the absence of data.

The published population-based epidemiological studies are summarized in Table 1. Pertinent details are included about the population (location, age, gender), dietary methodology employed, adjustment for covariables, relationship of sodium and potassium, and the direction of the relationship of calcium and blood pressure. Each study will be described and reviewed for consistency of relationship, the apparent independence of the calcium effect, potential interactions with and adjustment for critical covariables, and analytical differences that might clarify ambiguities and mechanisms and improve the focus of future research.

The data are derived from diverse populations throughout the industrialized world. The countries are from two continents, and include the United States (and Puerto Rico) and the Netherlands. The ethnic groups include Caucasian, Japanese, black, and Hispanic. There are no data from lesser-developed countries. An important difference between blood pressure studies of calcium and sodium is the analytical construct. The majority of studies that demonstrate a relationship between sodium and blood pressure depend on cross-cultural comparisons, usually across countries [22]. The reason is that wide differences in sodium intake are necessary to demonstrate blood pressure differences, and these wide variations are not usually found within most industrialized countries. On the other hand, the described relationship between calcium and blood pressure is found in comparisons within populations. Sufficient variation in calcium intake occurs within industrialized populations to find these associations. In general, observations within populations are likely to have greater therapeutic utility because there are groups within the social and cultural context who have achieved the beneficial behavior. Therefore, one could expect that a recommendation for change could be accomplished in this setting. Moreover, analyses within populations afford better opportunities to identify and to control or adjust for relevant covariables. This considerably strengthens the analysis.

The ages of the surveyed populations include adults aged 18 to 80 years (second column in Table 1) and both men and women. Blood pressure is

TABLE 1. Population Surveys Examining the Relationship Between Dietary Calcium and Blood Pressure

Population	Age/gender restriction	Relationship CA-BP	Adjusted	Relationship Na⁺ K⁺	Dietary measurment	Sample size
Oregon[3]		↓	Matched 1,7,8	None		90
Honolulu[4]	Japanese/American men 45–64	↓ bivariate	1,2	Na⁺ none	24-hr recall milk	6858
Rancho Bernardo[5]	Age 30–79	↓ Rx'd HTN women; ↓ SBP men	1,6,3		Whole milk Whole milk	5050 541 males
Rural Iowa[6]	Women 20–80	NS/Low vit D low Ca⁺⁺ sign	1,2,3,4,5	None	CA⁺⁺ H_2O food freq, 24-hr recall, diet 10 years ago	308
Western Electric[7]	Men 40–56	↓ DBP			28-day diet hx	1976
Puerto Rico[8]	Men 45–64	↓ urban; rural 55–64	1,3,10–17		24-hr recall milk	7932
Netherlands[9]	men DOB 1900–1919	↓ 1965 & 1970	1	↓ K⁺	Usual foods & alcohol	794 1960 605 1965 498 1970
Netherlands[10]	40–65	↓ SBP	1–4,10, 20–22	↓ Na⁺, K⁺		1,244 males 1,047 females
*NHANES-I[11]	25–74	↑ male SBP ↓ female DBP	1,2	↓ male DBP NA⁺/K⁺ ↓ K⁺	24-hr recall	996 males 1,059 females
NHANES-I[12]	18–74	↓ DBP males 21–74; female 21–55 HTN/NL	1,3,7,8 Stratified	↓ K⁺	24-hr recall	10,372
NHANES-II[13]	21–74	↓ females 21–74	1,2,6 18,19	None	24-hr recall freq CA⁺⁺ foods	Males* Females*

1 = age, 2 = BME, 3 = alchol intake, 4 = smoking, 5 = physical activity, 6 = age², 7 = race, 8 = gender, 9 = relative weight, 10 = pulse, 11 = cigarettes smoked, 12 = blood glucose, 13 = education, 14 = CHO, 15 = fat, 16 = protein, 17 = coffee, 18 = serum zinc, 19 = RBC, 20 = energy intake, 21 = serum cholesterol, 22 = hemoglobin.

*Number varies; all cases must be complete for variables selected.

positively correlated with age. In each survey, an adjustment was made for the age-related increase in blood pressure, and generally this was done through stratification or regression analysis or by the use of age-matched hypertensive and normotensive persons.

The relationship between dietary calcium and blood pressure is generally inverse (indicated by the downward arrow in the third column). The measures of blood pressure illustrating this relationship have included systolic pressure or diastolic pressure or classification as hypertensive/normotensive based on systolic/diastolic criteria. It should be noted that statistically significant relationships are demonstrated in some studies for either systolic or diastolic pressure or both. The relationship may be noted for one age or gender group, and this is noted in this column. There is not a clear preference for the association to be found for either systolic or diastolic pressure. The relationship to blood pressure has generally been found throughout the entire range of pressures and not just across an arbitrary separation between hypertensive-normotensive. This implies a more general physiological relationship between calcium intake and blood pressure and not an association between a "disease state"—hypertension—and a modified dietary intake. Moreover, modification of dietary intake or use of medications can follow diagnosis and obscure dietary relationships.

Dietary calcium intake can vary by age, race, body mass, and alcohol consumption. Various studies have attempted to control for the confounding effect of these variables. Most studies have controlled for age. This is especially important because blood pressure increases and calcium intake decreases with increased age. Several analyses controlled for age and body-mass index, while others controlled for many additional factors—i.e., physical activity, race, and sex. The adjustments of covariables are given for the various studies and indexed in the footnote to the table. Foods contain multiple nutrients, and there can be colinearity of nutrient intake that can confound relationships with blood pressure [23]. This has been noted for calcium and potassium. Racial patterns in eating and hypertension may also be confounding. Black persons have a higher prevalence of hypertension in the United States, but blacks consume less calcium on the average than do whites [20]. This is thought to be due to the high prevalence of lactose intolerance in black persons. Therefore, if race is not considered, an incorrect association may be found.

In one of the earliest descriptions of a difference in calcium intake in hypertension, Langford and Watson reported statistically significant differences in a survey of black persons in Mississippi [2]. The investigators had designed a study to test the hypothesis that racial differences in sodium and potassium intake were associated with the higher pressures in black persons. However, the sodium and potassium intakes did not differ across race or blood pressure. Calcium intake was lower in hypertensive persons. Few covariables were assessed, and there was no adjustment for weight or alcohol use.

A pilot study in Oregon matched 46 hypertensives by age, gender, and race to 44 normotensive controls and compared the intake of calcium [3]. Hypertensive subjects were not receiving antihypertensive medications. Mean age and body weights of the two groups did not differ. No differences were found for calories consumed or sodium and potassium intake. The calcium consumption differed significantly between the two groups. Only 8 of 46 hypertensives consumed more than 1 gm of calcium per day, compared to 18 of 44 normotensives whose intake was greater than 1 g/day. The difference in calcium consumption depended on the intake of dairy products other than milk. These sources provided 400 and 148 mg of calcium for normotensive and hypertensives, respectively.

Between 1972 and 1974, adults of Rancho Bernardo, an upper-class community in southern California, were surveyed for the Lipid Research Clinic study [5]. Data from individuals at the first visit had information about the consumption of whole milk. Young subjects (30 to 54 years old) consumed significantly more whole milk than older subjects, and men consumed significantly more than women. Consumption of whole milk was significantly lower in borderline treated and untreated hypertensive men than in normotensives. However, for women only, the treated hypertensives consumed significantly less calcium than normotensive women. For males, both systolic and diastolic blood pressure increased with decreasing calcium intake. The trend, after adjusting for age and obesity, was significant only for diastolic in men. Calcium from all dairy products was inversely correlated ($p < 0.05$) with diastolic blood pressure and whole milk with systolic blood pressure in males after adjusting for age, obesity, and alcohol consumption. Whole milk consumption was significantly and inversely correlated with alcohol consumption after controlling for age and obesity. The study collected no data on calcium intake from nondairy products.

Women from two rural communities in Iowa were studied for the effect of calcium on blood pressure [6]. These two communities were selected because of their water supplies. One community had an elemental calcium level of 375 mg/l and the other 65 mg/l in the water. Women were studied who had lived in their respective communities for at least 5 years prior to the study, and women using antihypertensives were excluded from the analyses. The investigators found no significant relationship between calcium intake and blood pressure either before or after adjusting for age, body-mass index, and alcohol consumption. Calcium values were calculated from food-frequency checklists or 24-hour recall. Intake of vitamin D was not normally distributed, so it was dichotomized at 400 IU. In young women, vitamin D was significant and inversely associated with systolic blood pressure after the inclusion of body-mass index, alcohol intake, and calcium. In older women (55 to 80 years), low vitamin D (<400 IU) and low calcium (<800 mg/day) were associated with a higher systolic blood pressure.

The Western Electric study used a 28-day diet history, which provides perhaps the most representative sampling of individual intake [7]. In this study, diastolic blood pressure was found to be positively correlated with age, body-mass index, and ethanol intake. Diastolic blood pressure was inversely associated with dietary calcium, monounsaturated fatty acids, and polyunsaturated fatty acids. The authors reported that, except for body-mass index, the associations were small, but statistically significant, for all nutrients.

The Puerto Rico Heart Program investigated the relationship between calcium and blood pressure in their population of men [18]. Men between the age of 45 and 64 who were free of coronary heart disease and not on antihypertensive medications at baseline were eligible for the study. Subjects were required to have completed a 24-hour diet recall to be included in the calcium–blood pressure analyses. There were 7,932 such men. The investigators found subjects who drank no milk had twice the prevalence of hypertension as men who drank a quart or more each day. There was an inverse trend between calcium consumptions and blood pressure. The relationship was seen in urban men aged 45 to 54 years and 55 to 64 years and rural men aged 55 to 64, years but not in the younger rural men. These relationships persisted after adjustment in multivariate analyses. The variables included were milk (4-oz. units/day), protein, fats, carbohydrates, coffee, alcohol, education, blood glucose, relative weight, pulse, cigarettes smoked per day, and age.

A random sample of males born between 1900 and 1919, residing in Zutphen, the Netherlands, were enrolled in 1960 in a longitudinal study of the relationship between diet, other risk factors, and chronic disease [9]. Eight hundred seventy-one males completed both the medical examination and the diet survey in 1960. The medical examinations and diet surveys were repeated in 1965 and 1970. Information on diet was collected on the usual food and alcohol consumption patterns during the 6 to 12 months prior to the survey. The mean intake of calcium was 1.2 gm/day. Potassium was inversely related to systolic blood pressure in 1970 and was of borderline significance in 1960 and 1970 in the multiple linear regression. Calcium was inversely related to systolic blood pressure and diastolic blood pressure in 1965 and 1970. The relationship persisted in the multiple linear regression with alcohol intake, energy intake, quetelets index, and age. However, changes in potassium and calcium intake during follow-up were not related to changes in blood pressure.

Analyses of another study conducted in the Netherlands in 1950 found calcium to be inversely related to blood pressure in a multiple linear regression model that included age, body-mass index, energy intake, serum cholesterol, smoking, alcohol consumption, hemoglobin, and pulse rate [10]. Sodium and potassium were also inversely related to blood pressure, although the association was not statistically significant in the multivariate analysis. Hypertensive males consumed 4.4% less calcium than normotensives, and hypertensive females consumed 5% less than their normotensive counterparts. No differences were seen between the groups as regards potassium or sodium intake.

Several analyses have been made of the U.S. national surveys and have provoked the greatest controversy [11–14]. An analysis of the National Health and Nutrition Examination Survey I (NHANES-I) used the detailed subsample of males and females not receiving antihypertensive medication to investigate systolic and diastolic blood pressures in multiple-regression models. NHANES-I was conducted from 1971 to 1974. It examined a representative sample of the U.S. population, and when the appropriate analytic framework is applied the findings can be considered representative of the entire U.S. population. Data suggested that dietary calcium was inversely and significantly related to diastolic blood pressure in a regression model for females, which also included age, body-mass index, pulse rate, serum phosphorus, serum urate, hemoglobin, and serum aspertate aminotransferase. In the final multiple-regression model for men, calcium was positively related to systolic blood pressure in the model with age, body-mass index, pulse rate, serum phosphorus, serum urate, and serum aspertate aminotransferase. No measure of sodium intake, or intake of salty foods or sodium content of foods, was related to blood pressure. There was a positive relationship between the Na^+/K^+ ratio in foods and diastolic blood pressure in males [11].

Another analysis of the NHANES-I data, using an unweighted statistical approach and another subset of individuals, investigated the relationship of 17 nutrients in 10,372 individuals aged 18 to 74 who had no history of hypertension, were not on a special diet, and were not pregnant [12]. Lower consumptions of calcium, potassium, vitamin A, and vitamin C were found when hypertensives, using several definitions of hypertension, were compared to normotensives after adjusting for age, gender, race, and body-mass index. The proportion of individuals with systolic blood pressures ≥ 160 mmHg increased with decreasing increments of dietary calcium. However, there was not an adjustment for age, race, or gender in that analysis and, as noted, this complex design of the survey requires statistical adjustment as well as consideration of sampling and response bias.

The NHANES-II (1976–80) data were used to investigate the relationship of blood lead and blood pressure [13]. Calcium intake using food-frequency patterns was inversely related to hypertension in the young group (21 to 55 years), but only for females in the 56–74-year-old group. Respondents on antihypertensive medications were included in analysis. In the multivariate analyses, dietary calcium was selected as an independent predictor of both systolic and diastolic blood pressure in females, but was not related to either in males. Blood leads were selected in the model for males. Calcium and lead are known to compete for absorption, excretion and, in the metabolic pathways, and the inclusion of one ion in the model may lead to the exclusion of the other, because of colinearity.

A recent analysis of NHANES-I and NHANES-II data by Sempos et al. concluded that there was no general relationship between low calcium intake and blood pressure [14]. These analyses incorporated appropriate statistical adjustments for design and sample weights and compared quintiles of calcium intake to explore gradients of effect as well as the relationship to those designated "hypertensive." There were adjustments for age and body-mass index (wt/ht^2). A significantly higher systolic and diastolic pressure was associated with lower calcium intake for black men in NHANES-I, and this agrees with the findings of Harlan et al. using different gender-race categories and multiple-regression analysis. The analysis by Sempos et al. did not find any significant relationship in NHANES-II in contrast to the reports by Harlan et al. The two analyses of NHANES-II differed in the exclusions from analysis. Sempos and colleagues excluded persons reporting "regular or occasional" use of antihypertensive agents, while Harlan and colleagues did not. This inclusion or exclusion of treated hypertensive individuals in analysis is an important undecided question. Public knowledge about hypertension and aggressive initiation of therapies have led to relatively high proportions of persons being treated either pharmacologically or nonpharmacologically. This proportion has increased progressively since the early 1970s, and the handling of survey data since this time will be biased depending on the handling of data for treated persons.

The risk of eliminating treated hypertensives from exploration of other relationships is that a major proportion of persons of greatest interest and at the end of a continuous distribution are lost to analysis. This will jeopardize the sample size in this critical category and imperil the ability to get stable estimates and detect significant differences. Alternatively, inclusion of persons on treatment might have conflicting effects. If the medication lowers blood pressure, this will blur the relationship, particularly if the treatment restores the pressure to normal. Also, dietary changes initiated in treatment (e.g., low salt or calcium augmentation) may obviate any differences present in the "natural" or untreated state or even reverse the direction of the relationship. As noted, this problem is becoming more important as treatment becomes more extensive and more effective. The effect is greater in

NHANES-II (1976–1980) than in NHANES-I (1971–1975), and this may explain the fading relationship in the Sempos et al. analyses.

There are several other issues that require comment in interpreting these studies. First, the studies deal exclusively with industrialized societies, and the dietary patterns in these populations are generally high in sodium, saturated fats, protein, and total calories, and relatively low in potassium. This background of dietary intake may be important in conditioning the physiological need and response to calcium. For example, calcium absorption is decreased and excretion increased with high protein intake. High sodium intake also enhances calcium excretion. Therefore, the calcium requirement may be greater in populations or segments of the population consuming high-protein, high-sodium diets. Many other nutrients also affect blood pressure and may be contained in the same foods or be incorporated into a particular eating pattern. Calcium and potassium contents are high in dairy products, and potassium intake, like that of calcium, has an inverse relationship with blood pressure. This makes it difficult to distinguish the blood pressure effects of each ion. Therefore, the dietary context of the populations can have an important modifying effect as well as a confounding effect on the relationship of dietary calcium to blood pressure. The relationship of calcium intake in nonindustrialized countries might be different with respect to both the existence of a relationship and the strength of the relationship. It would be of interest to explore the calcium–blood pressure relationship in populations whose intake is characterized as lower in calories, protein, and sodium and higher in potassium. This dietary intake characterizes many developing countries. Presumably, in this situation, the total requirement for calcium might be lessened, and it would be instructive to determine whether the calcium-intake effect persists.

The second issue is the appropriate adjustments for other nutrients when analysis is performed. There is no doubt that age, gender, and body mass (or adiposity) have important associations with blood pressure and must be treated as covariates with adjustment for their effect. The problem of adjustment for other nutrients is that they may vary colinearly with calcium [23]. Therefore, it may be difficult to determine which nutrient has the primary or more important association. This cannot be determined by the magnitude of the correlation or by the most tenable biological mechanism. The problem of calcium-potassium colinearity in the Japanese-Hawaiian population has been examined by Reed et al. [23]. They conclude that in this population dairy products are important sources of both calcium and potassium and lead to a high correlation between the two measurements. When each is regressed against blood pressure, it was not possible to assign a primary effect to either ion. The potassium intake from nondairy sources was also inversely related to blood pressure, and potassium appeared to be more closely related to blood pressure than calcium. In other populations with different dietary patterns, this same confounding of nutrients may not occur, but the general problem remains. Within populations, eating patterns tend to vary by social and educational strata, and food selection comprises a pattern of interrelated selections. Persons consuming dairy products may frequently consume fruits, leafy vegetables, and seafood, as well as moderate amounts of alcohol. To the degree that these food selections coexist for many persons and characterize a socioeconomic group, there will be confounding of the effect of single nutrients and of socioeconomic status on other measures, such as blood pressure. There is an advantage to having assessments in several populations with diverse dietary and social patterns. Consistency of a relationship with a specific nutrient when the food-consumption patterns differ helps to isolate the nutrients of primary importance.

These epidemiologic observations can be interpreted as indicating a fragile inverse relationship between dietary calcium and blood pressure. This relationship becomes less robust when adjustments are made for important co-variables such as age, gender, and body mass, and may be very dependent on the inclusion or exclusion of hypertensive persons or treatment. Moreover, secular trends in dietary intake of calcium, sodium, and other nutrients, as well as calcium supplementation, may further obscure the relationship in current and future surveys. The increasing dietary and drug treatment of hypertension may further blur a relationship in industrialized countries.

This calcium–blood pressure relationship should also be put in the context of other nutritional variables related to blood pressure. In all of the surveys, body mass or adiposity had the most robust relationship with systolic and diastolic pressure after age and race. When alcohol use was measured, this nutrient had a consistent relationship, although the type of relationship varied from J-shaped to directly linear. The strength of relationship between dietary calcium and blood pressure was distinctly lower and less robust than body mass or alcohol [11]. However, in most surveys, sodium intake had an even less robust relationship than calcium. On the other hand, dietary potassium or sodium/potassium had associations of the same or less strength and robustness as calcium. As commented on previously, the within-individual variability on dietary assessment may be responsible for the fragile and inconsistent dietary relationships.

Observational studies can be used as guides to planning interventional studies, but do no constitute adequate proof to recommend adaptation of a particular life-style or to add supplemental foods. These studies can indicate the levels at which intervention would be successful and suggest expected levels of change. From the observational studies, it would appear that levels of calcium intake above 800 to 1000 mg per day would be necessary to achieve a blood pressure effect. Moreover, to ensure that the effect could be

TABLE 2. Studies Using Calcium Supplementation to Lower Blood Pressure

Population	Restriction	Calcium supplement	Control	Trial length	Results	Sample size
Oregon[24]	unRx'd HTN	1.0 gm/day	—	4 years	Suppl. HTN ↓	115
Oregon[25]	Postmenopausal osteo study	1.0–1.2 gm/day	Match normotensives	8 weeks	MAP* ↓ p <.01	81
Wisconsin[26]	Women 35–64 yr	1.5 gm/day	—	2 years	↓ HTN suppl	70
Guatemala[27]	18–35 yr	1.0 gm/day	Placebo	22 weeks	↓ DBP+	57
Guatemala[28]	Pregnant 20–35 yr	1.0 & 2.0 gm/day	Placebo	23 weeks	↓ 2 Gm Ca²⁺ group	36
Netherlands[29]	Mild hypertensive 16–29 yr	1.0 gm/day	Placebo	12 weeks	↓ DBP+	90

*Mean arterial pressure.
+Diastolic blood pressure.

attributed to calcium, it would be preferable to supplement intake with elemental calcium rather than make dietary changes. Altering diet may lead to changes in other nutrients and confound the effect of calcium changes. In planning and evaluating interventions, it is clear that the effect of weight reduction and moderation of alcohol intake must be included, as these two factors can have important effects on blood pressure. Intervention trials can provide additional epidemiologic evidence regarding a calcium effect on blood pressure.

CALCIUM SUPPLEMENTATION STUDIES

Support for an effect of calcium intake on blood pressure is provided by several studies of calcium supplementation. The published studies are summarized in Table 2. A lowering of blood pressure in several groups has been reported in persons treated with supplemental calcium. A greater decrease in blood pressure was found for hypertensives, although some decrease was reported in normotensives as well.

In an 8-week randomized, double-blind calcium supplementation study of 39 untreated hypertensives and 31 matched normotensive controls, 1 gm per day of calcium decreased the mean pressure of hypertensives but did not alter blood pressure in normotensive persons [24]. Systolic blood pressure was reduced ($p < .05$), but diastolic blood pressure remained unchanged. Using as a definition of responsiveness a 10 mmHg decrease in pressure during supplementation, the mean change of the responders was 17 ± 8 mmHg and 18 ± 7 mmHg for the hypertensives and normotensives, respectively. Of the hypertensives, 42% were responders and 13% of the normotensives were responders.

Women 35 to 65 years of age were studied in a 4-year clinical trial to assess age-associated bone loss in women who did or did not receive supplemental calcium (1.0 to 1.5 g) [26]. Normotensive women had no significant change in blood pressure. Hypertensive women receiving supplemental calcium had a 13-mmHg drop in systolic blood pressure, and those not receiving calcium experienced a 7-mmHg rise during the 4 years. Hypertensive women tended to have lower (p = 0.07) average dietary calcium intake before supplementation. When two hypertensive women with high calcium intakes but not on supplementation were removed from the group, the difference in calcium intake was significant (p < 0.025). No relationship between blood pressure and calcium supplementation was observed for normotensive women, but there was also no age-related increase in blood pressure as might be expected over the 4 years. This study has special interest because of the long period of supplementation (4 years), the magnitude (13 mmHg) of mean blood pressure decrease in hypertensives, and the careful dietary assessment. No differences between supplemented and unsupplemented women were observed for changes in diastolic pressure, and there were no differences in caloric intake or dietary magnesium.

Belizan conducted a double-blind clinical trial of calcium supplementation in healthy adults 18 to 35 years of age [27]. The subjects, 28 men and 29 women, were not receiving any medical treatment at the time of recruitment, and women were not on oral contraceptives. In separate randomizations based on age categories, 18- to 23-year-old and 24- to 35-year-old subjects were assigned to supplementation of 1 gm of elemental calcium per day or placebo and the study design was double blind. Dietary intake, including dietary calcium, was also assessed. No dietary changes were seen in calories, protein, fat, iron, or calcium intake within or between groups, except for a significant decrease (p < 0.05) in dietary calcium among the calcium-supplemented men in the latter half of the study. During calcium supplementation, both men and women had a statistically significant decrease in systolic blood pressure and diastolic blood pressure. The decreases in blood pressure were generally in the range of 3% to 10%. The decrease in blood pressure occurred in 3 to 6 weeks, and the resulting pressure was stable in the 6th and 9th weeks for men and women, respectively, indicating a rather rapid onset of effect.

A follow-up supplementation study was conducted in 36 women enrolled during the second trimester of their pregnancy [28]. The women were randomized to one of three treatment groups: placebo, 1 gm/day calcium supplementation, and 2 gm/day calcium supplementation. The groups did not differ at baseline with respect to calcium intake, demographics, or clinical variables. Dietary intake was assessed using a 24-hour recall method. The placebo group's blood pressures "oscillated" throughout the pregnancy. Both calcium-supplemented groups had reductions in systolic blood pressure in the second trimester. After the 26th and 32nd week, the 1 gm/day and the placebo groups experienced an increase in their systolic blood pressure. The 2 gm group had no increase in blood pressure, and levels remained significantly lower than those for either the 1 gm or the placebo group. The parathyroid hormone, while not significantly different, tended to be lower at the 38th week of gestation in the 2 gm group in contrast to the increase seen in the placebo group. There was a significant partial correlation coefficient ($r = .30$) between initial parathyroid hormone levels and diastolic pressure.

In a double-blind trial in the Netherlands, Grobbee and Hofman administered 1.0 gm per day of elemental calcium to 90 (77 male) mildly hypertensive persons aged 16 to 29 years [29]. This is a particularly interesting group because of their relatively young age, a 7- to 9-year follow-up with frequent blood pressures over 140/90 mmHg prior to study, and the relevance for nonpharmacologic treatment of young hypertensives. The group receiving calcium supplementation experienced a decrease in seated diastolic blood pressure (3.1 mmHg at 6 weeks and 2.4 at 12 weeks) when compared with the placebo control group. Subjects complying with therapy had greater declines in pressure (5.1 mmHg and 3.9 mmHg). Small and nonsignificant differences were found in systolic. When analyzed by baseline characteristics, the blood pressure responsiveness was confined to those with parathyroid hormone levels above the group median, and the decline in diastolic pressure was significantly associated with a decrease in parathyroid hormone levels. These observations lend credence to the view that blood pressure responsiveness to calcium supplementation can be identified prior to therapy and may be linked to regulation of parathyroid hormone secretion.

Review of these studies suggests that there is a difference in individual responsiveness to supplemental calcium. McCarron suggested there were calcium responders and nonresponders [24], suggesting an analogy to blood pressure responsiveness to sodium restriction. A randomized placebo-controlled trial using a supplement of 1.5 gm/day showed a significant decrease in mean arterial pressure compared to placebo [30]. He characterized the responders based on a 10 mmHg or greater response. Within the calcium-supplemented group, responders were older and had higher baseline mean arterial pressures, higher baseline parathyroid hormone, and lower baseline serum total calcium. Grobbee and Hofman [29], who studied young adults, also characterized responders as having higher baseline parathyroid hormone levels. Discriminant function analysis correctly classified 78.8% of the responders and nonresponders using mean arterial pressure and serum total calcium. These determinants of responsiveness are important. A large-scale trial would need independent pretrial measures of responsiveness to ensure an adequate test of efficacy of calcium supplementation.

The results of calcium-supplementation studies share some similarities, but there are other troublesome differences. Dietary intake of calcium prior to supplementation was generally below the RDA and in the range of 500 to 600 mg/day for most groups studied. Therefore, addition of 1000 to 1500 mg per day represented a repair of inadequate intake as well as a supplement above recommended levels. Although there was an apparent dose-response relationship in pregnant women who had a greater daily requirement, this was not observed in others. This suggests that a dose of 1000 to 1500 mg in the nonpregnant state is adequate to obtain a therapeutic response. This would be added to dietary intake of 600 to 800 mg to yield 1600 to 2300 mg per day intake. Although this exceeds the current RDA, there is some evidence that the RDA is defined at a lower than optimal level. The blood pressure lowering effect is established within 6 to 8 weeks and is stable by 16 weeks. The effect persists for at least 4 years based on the single long-term study. Further studies of extended calcium supplementation are needed, and additional studies are needed to determine of the minimum period necessary to achieve a stable blood pressure reduction in those who respond. At least one negative trial of 4 weeks may not have been continued sufficiently long to observe a response [31]. Two other trials have reported in abstracts that no blood pressure lowering occurred, but insufficient data prevent evaluation [32,33].

The blood pressure response to short-term supplementation was modest and was found more often for systolic than for diastolic pressures. More importantly, the calcium-supplementation effect was consistently greater in hypertensive persons than in those with normal pressures, and often there were no significant changes in normotensive persons. The studies of Belizan et al. contrast with the others in this regard [27]. They found significant decreases in diastolic pressures in healthy, normotensive adults and in normotensive pregnant women. The long-term study of middle-aged women found a large reduction of systolic pressure (13 mmHg) in hypertensive women, but no change in diastolic pressure. The reason for the difference in findings is not obvious, but diastolic pressure varies within a narrower range than systolic, and measurement of diastolic pressure is more difficult. This tends to minimize the ability to find changes from therapeutic maneuvers that exceed observer and within-individual variability. Future studies should direct attention to standardization of blood pressure observation, and random-zero syphmomanometers may assist in overcoming digit preference. The position of the subject when blood pressure is recorded may be important. McCarron found decreases in standing pressures, but not in sitting or supine [30]. Belizan reported the greatest changes in diastolic pressure in the dorsal position and least in the seated position [27]. In the Dutch study of young adults, sitting diastolic pressures decreased by not systolic. This study used random-zero syphmonometers and thereby decreased observer bias. The differences may relate to measurement technique or timing and sequence of examination procedures. It is clear that future studies should record pressures in several positions and probably multiple pressures in each position. The clinical convention of recording seated pressures may miss an important effect of calcium supplementation.

Another issue in calcium-supplementation studies relates to the diet content preceding and during supplementation. Is the calcium that is taken a replacement for a diet inadequate in calcium—that is, correcting a deficiency? If this represents a replacement, then differential results might be expected depending on the dietary status of the individual. The diets in the U.S. and most industrialized countries are relatively high in salt and protein, and low in potassium and magnesium. This typical diet increases the requirement for calcium intake to maintain an adequate balance of total body calcium. Moreover, the typical diet includes less than the recommended daily allowance (RDA) for calcium. The calcium "supplement" may be only a replacement for inadequate intake. The interaction of calcium with other dietary constituents is critical. For example, individuals who are on a diet modest in salt or protein content or a diet with increased potassium intake may not respond as well to increased calcium intake. On the other hand, a high salt intake may create a physiological setting that maximizes blood pressure lowering with supplemental calcium.

Responsiveness is important in assessing either calcium supplementation or sodium restriction. With either maneuver, about half will respond with a biologically and statistically significant fall in pressure. No one has examined whether the same individuals are responsive to the sodium and calcium interventions. Calcium "responders" are characterized as having higher entry blood pressures (i.e., hypertensive), being older in age, having higher baseline parathyroid hormone, and having lower serum-ionized calcium [34]. Interestingly, these characteristics, except the lower serum calcium, are those that might be expected from inadequate dietary intake or from use of diuretic medication. This suggests that "responders" may designate individuals who have an inadequate calcium intake in the dietary context of this country.

A related issue is the utility of calcium supplementation when other dietary approaches to hypertension are being used. Sodium restriction and weight reduction are currently accepted as the most promising nonpharmacologic approaches to mild hypertension or prevention of hypertension in susceptible individuals. What is the efficacy of calcium supplementation with sodium restriction, and is there an additive effect of the two approaches? Weight reduction is perhaps the most potent nonpharmacologic approach to

TABLE 3. Issues for Future Calcium-Supplementation Trials

Design:	Randomized, placebo controlled with minimum of 20 weeks treatment period. Double blin preferable.
Subjects:	Probable "responder"—i.e., older (>50 years of age) men or women with mild hypertensive pressures (systolic 140–160 mmHg and/or diastolic 90–100 mmHg) and not on medication or sodium restriction. Adequate sample size to detect 8 mmHg systolic or 4 mmHg diastolic.
Intervention:	Elemental calcium containing 1 gm per day.
Measurements:	1) Preceding and concurrent diet and supplemental intake of vitamins and minerals assessed with special attention to sodium, potassium, magnesium, calcium and vitamin D. 2) Blood pressures seated and standing (2 to 3 each) at biweekly intervals with observers standardized and blinded to treatment. 3) Weight, alcohol intake, and activity maintained constant.

hypertension. Does blood pressure respond to calcium supplementation during weight reduction or the maintenance period after weight reduction? These interrelationships require investigation to define the role of calcium supplementation in therapy, given that it will compete for acceptance with two better-established modes of therapy. Based on the foregoing discussion, several important features can be proposed for future studies of calcium supplementation and are listed in Table 3.

MECHANISMS

Epidemiological studies usually are not directed toward identifying or clarifying physiological mechanisms, but often they can identify important relationships that afford clues to mechanisms. In the broad view of the dietary relationship of calcium and blood pressure, several aspects stand out. First, the physiological distance between dietary intake and the presumed cellular action is immense. The intermediary link, the extracellular calcium concentration, is defended rigorously against wide excursions regardless of dietary intake. This defense involves interaction of several identified hormones and depends on modulation of bone buildup and breakdown and on changes in renal excretion. It seems unlikely that variations in dietary calcium could directly vary extracellular concentrations or events related to cellular metabolism. It seems more likely that other, less direct mechanisms are responsible. Several mechanisms can be proposed that could direct appropriate data collection in field studies and trials.

First, the relative deficiency of calcium consumed and absorbed or excessive excretion might lead to a decrease in calcium balance and to com-

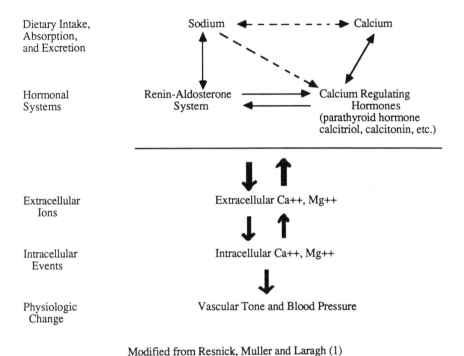

Modified from Resnick, Muller and Laragh (1)

Fig. 1. Hypothetical scheme linking dietary intake to hormonal regulation and extra- and intra-cellular changes.

pensatory hormonal changes. These hormonal changes, in turn, mediate blood pressure changes. Clinical observations and studies indicate that calcium-regulating hormones (parathyroid calcitonin and calcitriol) can alter vascular tone and blood pressure. Calcium-regulating hormones have, in turn, been related to sodium-regulating hormones by Resnick and co-workers [1,35].

A hypothetical scheme presented by Resnick has been modified and is shown in Figure 1 [1]. The scheme is a conceptual construct of relationships and interactions and is not intended to suggest the primacy of a particular event, such as changes in dietary calcium. As noted in the diagram, calcium balance, including changes in intake, absorption, and excretion, can induce changes in the levels of the calcium-regulating hormones. These, in turn, have modulating effects on the salt-regulating hormones, renin and aldosterone. Parathyroid hormone varies inversely with plasma renin level but directly enhances aldosterone secretion. Serum calcitriol also varies inversely with plasma renin activity. The physiological and metabolic consequences of these hormonal changes are beyond the purview of this review and are shown merely to complete the picture. The hormonal changes can alter extracellular ion concentrations and intracellular ion movement, and these intracellular changes can lead to changes in vascular tone and blood pressure. There may also be more direct vasomotor effects of hormones.

This scheme indicates the important interactions between calcium intake and sodium intake. First, it should be appreciated that high dairy intake generally carries with it a relatively high sodium intake and the converse may have therapeutic implications. A low-sodium diet (75 mEq/day) requires restriction of dairy products and calcium. The excretion of calcium is dependent on salt balance, with high sodium intake enhancing calcium excretion. Moreover, parathyroid hormone levels are directly related to sodium excretion and may increase sodium retention when elevated. This indicates a hormonal mechanism by which calcium balance and parathyroid hormone may modulate sodium balance. Extracellular ion concentrations of calcium and magnesium can lead to changes in both the renin-aldosterone and the calcium-regulating systems.

These complex interactions occur at several levels of metabolism that can be assessed in future epidemiologic studies. It is clear that sodium balance must be considered in assessment of the role of calcium in changing blood pressure, whether such assessment is observational or interventional [36,37]. Secondly, measurement of calcium-regulating hormones and extracellular ionized calcium and magnesium can further expand the search for associations with blood pressure and mechanisms of action, although expensive, selective measurements in particular situations could be valuable. Future observations will alter and perhaps expand the hypothetical scheme, but it represents a framework for current understanding and for planning of other studies.

THERAPEUTIC IMPLICATIONS

There is clinical epidemiological evidence from observational and interventional studies to support an inverse relationship between calcium intake and blood pressure. The effect of calcium intake is apparently modest, and supplementation does not have a universal blood pressure lowering effect. This does not broadcast a clarion call to prevent or treat hypertension by increasing calcium intake or use of supplements. The effect is too variable among individuals and modest in degree. There is the other potential benefit of increasing dietary calcium, and that is increasing bone density. The RDA for calcium is not achieved by many persons, particularly the elderly, and the intake levels associated with elevated blood pressures lie within the zone of inadequate intake. It has been noted that the RDA may have been set at an inadequate level in our dietary context. Therefore, a clear recommendation can be made that the current RDA be achieved and that the current level be reassessed. This will require either increased dietary calcium or pill supplementation. Increasing calcium in the diet through increased use of dairy products has certain disadvantages that can be overcome. Dairy products carry high saturated fat and caloric content, but the use of skim milk and reduced-fat cheeses and ice milks effectively overcomes these disadvantages. There are an increasing number of food products processed so as to contain supplemental calcium, and these are being marketed aggressively. Manufacturers of vitamin and mineral supplements are increasing their interest in providing more calcium in the tablets. Whether these initiatives will provide adequate calcium intake will await current surveys of individual diet intake, such as the third National Health and Nutrition Examination Survey (NHANES-III).

The therapeutic use of calcium supplementation specifically in treatment of hypertension cannot be recommended now. Future trials are required to determine effectiveness and to compare the effectiveness of calcium supplementation with those of weight reduction, alcohol restriction, and sodium restriction. Calcium supplementation deserves further trials based on the present data and because of its simplicity and other potential benefits.

ACKNOWLEDGMENTS

Supported by NIH Grant HL 33407 and Diabetes Research Training Grant NIH AM 07445.

REFERENCES

1. Resnick LM, Muller FB, Laragh JH (1986): Calcium regulating hormones in essential hypertension: Relation to plasma renin activity and sodium metabolism. Ann Intern Med 105:649–654.
2. Langford HG, Watson RL (1973): Electrolytes, environment and blood pressure. Clin Sci Mol Med 45:1115–1135.
3. McCarron D, Morris CD, Cole C (1982): Dietary calcium in human hypertension. Science 217:267–69.
4. Reed D, McGee D, Yano K (1982): Biological and social correlates of blood pressure among Japanese men in Hawaii. Hypertension 4:406–14.
5. Ackley S, Barrett-Connor E, Suarez L (1983): Dairy products, calcium and blood pressure. Am J Clin Nutr 38:457–61.
6. Sowers MR, Wallace RB, Lemke JH (1985): The association of intakes of vitamin D and calcium with blood pressure among women. Am J Clin Nutr 42:135–142.
7. Nichaman M, Shekelle R, Paul O (1984): Diet, alcohol, and blood pressure in the Western Electric Study. Am J Epid 120:469–470.

8. Garcia-Palmieri MR, Costos R, Cruz-Vidal M, Sarlie PD, Tillston J, Havlik RJ (1984): Milk consumption, calcium intake, and decreased hypertension in Puerto Rico. Hypertension 6:322–28.

9. Kromkaut D, Bosschieter EB, de Lezenna Coulander C (1985): Potassium, calcium, alcohol intake and blood pressure: The Zutphen study. Am J Clin Nutr 41:1299–1304.

10. Kok FJ, Vandenkroucke, Van der Heide-Wessel C, Van der Heide RM (1986): Dietary sodium, calcium, potassium and blood pressure. Am J Epidemiol 123:1043–1048.

11. Harlan WR, Hull AL, Schmouder RL, Landis JR, Thompson FE, Larkin FA (1984): Blood pressure and nutrition in adults. The National Health and Nutrition Examination Survey. Am J Epidemiol 120:17–28.

12. McCarron DA, Morris CD, Henry HJ, Stanton JL (1984): Blood pressure and nutrient intake in the United States. Science 224:1393–1398.

13. Harlan WR, Landis JR, Schmounder RL, Goldstein NG, Harlan LC (1985): Blood lead and blood pressure: Relationship in the adolescent and adult U.S. population. JAMA 253:530–534.

14. Sempos C, Cooper R, Kovar MG, Johnson C, Drizd T, Yetley E (1986): Dietary calcium and blood pressure in National Health and Nutrition Examination Surveys I and II. Hypertension 8:1067–1074.

15. Kaplan NM, Meese RB (1986): The calcium deficiency hypothesis of hypertension: A critique. Ann Int Med 105:947–955.

16. Chu SY, Kolonel LN, Hankin JH, Lee J (1984): A comparison of frequency and quantitative dietary methods for epidemiologic studies of diet and disease. Am J Epidemiol 119:323–334.

17. Dietary Intake Source Data, United States, 1971–74, DHEW Publ. No. 79–1221, 1979.

18. Eaton SB, Konner M. Paleolithic nutrition (1985): A consideration of its nature and current implications. New Engl J Med 312:283–289.

19. Lakshamanan FL, Rao RB, Church JP (1984): Calcium and phosphorus intakes, balances, and blood levels of adults consuming self-selected diets. Am J Clin Nutr 40:1368–1379.

20. Lutwak L (1974): Dietary calcium and reversal of bone demineralization. Nutr News 37:1–4.

21. Pao EM (1981): Changes in American food consumption patterns and their nutritional significance. Food Technol 35:42–53.

22. Harlan WR, Harlan LC (1986): Dietary electrolytes and hypertension. J of Hypertension. 4:S334–39.

23. Reed D, McGee D, Yano K, Hankin J (1985): Diet, blood pressure, and multicollinearity. Hypertension 7:405–10.

24. McCarron DA, Henry HJ, Morris CD (1984): Randomized, placebo-controlled trial of oral Ca^{2+} in human hypertension. Clin Res 32:37A.

25. McCarron DA, Chestnut CH, Cole C, Baylink DJ (1981): Blood pressure response to the pharmacologic management of osteoporosis. Clin Res 29:274A.

26. Johnson NE, Smith EL, Freudenkeim JL (1985): Effects on blood pressure of calcium supplementation of women. Am J Clin Nutr 42:12–17.

27. Belizan JM, Villar J, Pineda O, Gonzalez AE, Sarnz NG, Garrera G, Sikrian R (1983): Reduction of blood pressure with calcium supplementation in young adults. JAMA 249: 1161–5.

28. Belizan JM, Villar J, Zalazar A, Rojas L, Chan D, Bryce GF (1983): Preliminary evidence of the effect of calcium supplementation on blood pressure in normal women. Am J Obstet Gynecol 146:175–80.

29. Grobbee DE, Hofman A (1986): Effect of calcium supplementation on diastolic blood pressure in young people with mild hypertension. Lancet 2:703–707.

30. McCarron DA, Morris CD (1985): Blood pressure response to oral calcium in persons with mild to moderate hypertension. Ann Int Med 103:825–831.

31. Meese RB, Gonzalez DG, Casparian JM, Ram CV, Pak CY, Kaplan NM (1986): Failure of calcium supplements to relieve hypertension. Clin Res 34:218A (abstract).

32. Strazzullo P, Siani A, Galletti F, et al. (1985): A controlled clinical trial of long term oral calcium supplementation in arterial hypertension (Abstract #512). In: ''Program of the 2nd European Meeting on Hypertension.'' Milan: University of Milan p. 213.

33. Singer DR, Markandu ND, Cappuccio FP, et al. (1985): Does oral calcium lower blood pressure: a double-blind study. J. Hypertens 3:661–71.

34. Grobbee DE, Hofman A (1986): Effect of calcium supplementation on diastolic blood pressure in young people with mild hypertension. Lancet 2:703–7.

35. Resnick LM, Laragh JH, Sealey JE, Alderman MN (1983): Divalent cations in essential hypertension: relations between serum ionized calcium, magnesium, and plasma renin activity. N Engl J Med 309:888–91.

36. Resnick LM, Case DB, Pickering TG (1983): The effect of dietary sodium loading on divalent ions in hypertension. Kidney Int 23:109 (abstract).

37. Resnick LM, Nicholson JP, Laragh JH (1985): Alterations in calcium metabolism mediate dietary salt sensitivity in essential hypertension. Trans Assoc Am Physicians 98:313–21.

Index